Stories in Ageing:
Reflection, Inquiry, Action

Second Edition

Stories in Ageing: Reflection, Inquiry, Action

Edited by Margaret Webb, Jan Skinner and Lisa Woodman

Second Edition

ELSEVIER

ELSEVIER

Elsevier Australia. ACN 001 002 357
(a division of Reed International Books Australia Pty Ltd)
Tower 1, 475 Victoria Avenue, Chatswood, NSW 2067

ISBN: 978-0-7295-4393-4

National Library of Australia Cataloguing-in-Publication Data

 A catalogue record for this book is available from the National Library of Australia

Senior Content Strategist: Melinda McEvoy
Content Project Manager: Shubham Dixit
Edited by Leanne Poll
Proofread by Tim Learner
Cover and internal design by Georgette Hall
Typeset by Toppan Best-set Premedia Limited
Printed in Singapore by Markono Print Media Pte Ltd

Author photographs courtesy of Meaghan Skinner

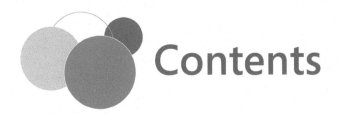

Contents

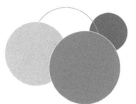

About the authors

Margaret Webb is a Registered Nurse with many years of experience within both the vocational and higher education sectors. She has a passion for curriculum design and the promotion of excellence in developing training materials. Her written works on the aged care and nursing sectors are well sought after and used throughout the health sectors in both Australia and New Zealand.

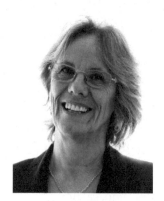

Jan Skinner is a Registered Nurse, educator, manager and researcher. She has worked in both the vocational education and university sectors, as well in the non-government sector managing nursing, non-nursing and allied health staff within a range of community services; caring for frail aged clients and those living with dementia; and providing services that facilitate reablement, support/maintenance and client choice. She also participates in research into ageing, dementia and nutrition in the older Australian, acting as an advisor on ageing within the tertiary and healthcare sectors.

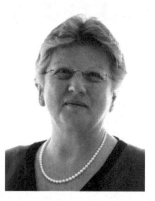

Lisa Woodman is a Registered Nurse, lecturer, consultant and researcher. She has worked extensively in aged care, including roles as a Director of Nursing, Chief Executive and aged care accreditor/advisor, and has managed hospitals and community services. She has been involved in both university undergraduate and post-graduate education as well as vocational education sector programs, and has worked as a consultant in Australia and Asia. She has a passion for ensuring quality of life in the older person, and assisting with empowerment of carers and family members. She also spends a great deal of time on promoting authentic holistic care for the person with dementia and helps international students gain transferrable knowledge.

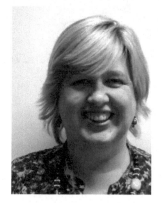

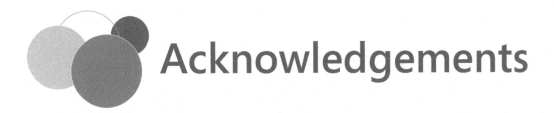

Acknowledgements

The authors would like to acknowledge all those who contributed to the development of this resource. For those who shared their stories and experiences with us, we are most grateful. It is only by listening and learning from those who hold knowledge and have 'lived experience' in the field of ageing that it is possible to gain a real understanding of ageing.

Helen Andrews

Lorna Annakin

Odette Best

Roseanne Birmingham

Maureen Brady

Barbara Berglind

Ali Drummond

Theresa Harvey

Brendan Horsfield

Lachlan Horsfield

Dawn Jen

Cindy Jones

Wendy Kane

Larry Loveday

Judy McCrow

Leonie McDonald

Carole Meyer

Anne Otter

Rafael Pacheco

Ron Prescott

Sandy Robins

Anna Rogers

Mercedes Sepulveda

Robert Thie

Theodore Thie

Barbara Young

Shirley Watson

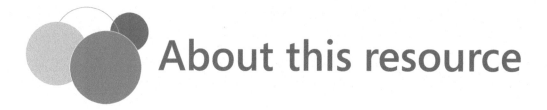

About this resource

Overview

This resource has been written specifically to present knowledge of ageing within a person-centred and lived approach. As it is based on actual experiences and real-life scenarios, the stories told reflect personal experiences rather than examples of the development of knowledge visualised through a theoretical lens.

The aim of this book is to engage the reader and link presented theories and practices to their actual application and impact on the person's experience. This resource focuses on the emotions and feelings that come from the participants talking about their experience.

It is also designed to assist learning in a manner that mirrors the way that we learn in everyday life: we listen to what we are told; we reflect on what we are told; we explore our options and reflections; and, finally, we develop a new or better understanding about what we know.

Using the resource

This resource is multilayered and is designed to engage learners from across a number of levels. It is not only suitable for students undertaking certificate-level qualifications, but also for those undertaking undergraduate-level degrees and completing post-graduate studies.

For those students requiring a more structured approach to learning, it can be used as a teaching tool with a teacher guiding the student/s through each section, working with them to gain an understanding of the ideas and theories presented.

Within the higher education sector, it can be used to facilitate a more exploratory approach to learning, with the instructor using the sections to prompt learning.

For those undertaking post-graduate studies, this resource can be used as a tool to identify areas of theory and/or practice which they may wish to explore in greater depth. The stories also offer greater potential as the foundation for future research.

This resource has a cross-disciplinary approach, allowing it to be used as a teaching/learning tool within a number of disciplinary areas in the health sector. Students in nursing, aged care and most allied health areas will find this resource useful and informative in contributing to their body of required knowledge. It may also be used within the clinical area for new graduates as a resource to guide their practice.

It is anticipated that this resource will be used online, by watching and listening to the videos and undertaking the activities online, or in hard copy format using the workbook and the stories written as transcripts.

Structure of the resource

There are a number of structures within this resource that are repeated within each chapter.

THE STORIES

Storytelling is a powerful way of learning and one which has been used throughout the centuries and across most cultural groups. It is a traditional way of passing on knowledge. Storytelling engages the listener, provides a context for the data and evokes images for the words, all of which promotes an authentic learning experience.

When we hear a story, we are likely to retain the embedded data much more efficiently than when we are told the same data in separate, unrelated chunks. The data is linked to actual events and experiences rather than presented as simply pieces of factual data. Listening to somebody tell their story also humanises that data, increasing our ability to personalise our practice and link it more efficiently to the 'lived experience' of our clients/residents.

Stories can also promote time for personal reflection for the listener to consider their own stories. Reflective practice is included as a component of the activities within each chapter, as it is an essential part of the learning process.

These are stories from actual people. They are not composite experiences put together to demonstrate a position or argument. These are real and factual experiences that each of the storytellers have experienced or have an in-depth understanding about. This authenticity gives the resource validity for the learner.

Each chapter focuses on a specific key understanding which is identified within the chapter heading. Within each chapter are a number of headings including Reflection, Inquiry and Action.

As the learner begins each chapter, prompts will direct the learner to view the story and then progressively work through the subheadings.

REFLECTION

The learner is asked to think about what they have listened to and make some personal judgment on this information. There are a number of questions that will help with this process and guide key learnings. This section is useful for learners at all levels.

INQUIRY

This section has been written to help the learner consider what else they need to know as well as identify any gaps in the knowledge presented that needs to be considered and any potential solutions.

ACTION

This is divided into three sections: **A**, **B** and **C**.

Within this section, the learner is invited to apply their knowledge and understandings to not only their personal practice but also to the organisational and political frameworks in which their practice is embedded.

This section has been organised within a stepping-up framework:

A generally asks the learner to apply their knowledge within the boundaries of their own personal practice.

B starts to introduce the notions of action within an organisational structure.

C generally asks for the knowledge gained to be applied within the greater political framework.

It should be noted that:

A will be better focused for the certificate-level learner

B is more for the undergraduate learner

C is intended to stimulate inquiry for the post-graduate learner.

This provides all learners with the opportunity to consolidate their foundational understandings of the data presented before moving on to the more complex concepts identified at the next level. Learners are able to advance to the next area if they wish and consider the learnings from these notions.

REFERENCES AND FURTHER READING

Bogossian, F 2005 Storytelling, concept mapping and reflection: a case study of an innovative teaching and learning approach to promote critical thinking about professional issues. Focus on health professional education: a multidisciplinary approach 7(1).

Lehmann, J 2003 Practice based stories: tools for teaching and learning. Children Australia. 28(1): 29–33.

Sriram, S n.d. Practice-based stories: a pedagogical tool in higher education. Brain Space. The Royal Melbourne Hospital. Available at: www.rmh.mh.org.au/story-telling-in-higher-education/w1/i1031802/

CHAPTER 1

Perspectives on Ageing

INTRODUCTION

This introductory chapter will help you understand how ageing and being an older person is perceived, from a cross-generational perspective. The stories in this chapter come from a panel of people comprised of a number of different age groups. The youngest panel member is 12 years old and the oldest is 66. While we are unable to develop a scientific analysis from such a small representation, the comments do provide some insight on how ageing is perceived as we move through the life span.

Before you begin ... How generational differences influence perceptions of ageing

Before you begin, think about your own views of what age you consider is old, ageing and the ageing experience. How do your perceptions reflect who you are and what your experiences have been? The following are some questions you should ask yourself.

1. Do you consider yourself old?
2. What age is old?
3. What are older people like?
4. What should older people not do?
5. What happens as people get older?
6. What makes a person old?
7. How would you personally know when you are old?
8. What would your generation be like when they are old?
9. Who should be responsible for the care of the older person?

These are the same questions that each of the panel members was asked to consider.

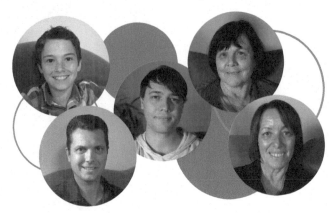

The Panel

View the panel's discussion or read the transcript.

Reflection

As you consider what the panel members have said, reflect on your own ideas and perceptions of who is considered to be an older person.

- Who is old?
- Are you old?
- What does ageing and being old mean to you?
- Which age group best aligns with your thoughts?
- Does the way that we perceive the older person influence the way that we undertake care within our practices?

What is old?

This question can have many different answers, In this text, we have tried not to put a definitive number on what is old. Consider the responses from the panel, defining the age as anything from 18 to 70 years old. They all qualify their answers with a reason for the age they see is old. There is no standard number that equates to being old. Helen, a 50-year-old panellist, also states:

> *I don't think you can really put an age on old. Like Theo said, some people are old at 30, there are people at 90 years old that really aren't old. I think it all depends on where you are and what stage you are in your life.*

If we consider how we are deemed to be old by government legislation we, find the following examples.

65 aged pension can be received (Australia)

60 seniors card can be received (Australia)

64–67 retirement age, depending on your gender and year of birth (Australia)

50 National Aboriginal and Torres Strait islander Flexible Aged Care Program (Australia)

85 and over elderly service age group (Brisbane Local Government Authority)

70–84 senior service age group (Brisbane Local Government Authority)

60 retirement age (Hong Kong)

65 old age allowance (Hong Kong)

65 retirement age for men (United Kingdom)

60 retirement age for women (United Kingdom)

62 early retirement (United States)

65–67 full retirement (United States)

If we consider the age of an older person to be the age when we are legally entitled to leave the workforce and enter retirement, you will see that there is no standardised definition or consensus on what chronological age is to be considered old. Plus, the services/entitlements available to a person who is old also vary.

A common theme you may see within the Panel story is that any definition of old or being an older person is always older than how a person sees themself. For example, 66-year-old panellist Anne could be classified as being old according to the above definitions; however, she did not put a number on 'being old' and just stated that 'we slow down a bit after the age of 70'. She does not see herself as being old.

Readings

Pause at this moment and complete the following readings. They will give you an overview on what is thought to be old.

When does old age begin?

http://seniorliving.about.com/od/agingwithattitude/a/when_does_old_age_begin.htm

Definition of an older or elderly person

www.who.int/healthinfo/survey/ageingdefnolder/en/

Definition of old age

www.info.gov.hk/gia/general/201103/02/P201103010256.htm

Old people feel 13 years younger than they are

www.livescience.com/3103-people-feel-13-years-younger.html

Sam Bryant, a 70-year-old bodybuilder

www.news.com.au/lifestyle/health/yearold-bodybuilder-sam-bryant-shows-age-isa-state-of-mind/story-fneuzle5-1226827853833

Reflection

Now reflect on what you have learned from the chapter so far.

- Do you recognise that there is a diverse range of numerical values placed on what it is to be considered an older person?

- Have your views on ageing changed in any way?

Inquiry

How we define an older person varies between countries, geopolitical boundaries and over time. While we would like to agree that it is based on the functionality, abilities and any number of other holistic attributes that make a person seem older, in reality the current economic and political situations more often dictate at what age a person is deemed to be old. If we link the age of retirement to be somewhat close to an age of being older, where once a woman was deemed old enough to retire and receive a pension at age 60, she must now wait until between the ages of 64 and 67 (depending on her year of birth).

Is this the most appropriate way of measuring age?

Action

A Consider how you would ensure within your clinical practice that you did not use stereotyped and preconceived perceptions of what age is old. What are some of the more practical things that you might do?

B Review the responses by each of the panellists and reflect on their answers to the questions: 'Do you consider yourself old?' and 'What age is old?' Try and determine why each of the panellists answered the way they did. What do you think was the reasoning behind each of the panellists' responses?

C Considering the legislative changes that have affected notions of what age is considered old, how have national and state politics set the age? How do national demographics and national and global economics affect the determination of what is the age of old? To answer this question we need

to assume that the national government's classification of an older person is linked to retirement and aged pensionable ages.

How should we determine what is old?

Does an individual have to go through an ageing process to be classed as old? Is there a set of rules and/or steps that a person has to pass through to be deemed old? From a scientific perspective senescence, which is the biological term for the ageing process, consists of a number of changes which are mostly degenerative. Physically, ageing commences at the cellular level and gradually affects the ultimate functioning of the body; our senses begin to dull, movements are less coordinated and body systems less efficient. Is this all that happens as we go through the ageing process? Do we succumb to a series of degenerative changes? Or is it more than that?

If we subscribe to a pure biological level of ageing then we need to agree with this, but if we pursue a more holistic viewpoint as did our panellists then we need to review this idea more. Brandon, the 44-year-old panellist, describes how he finds it difficult to identify who is old because of the way the older person looks and acts.

Ageing is much more than growing old physically. It is also to do with the way we think and act and the way in which we perceive ourselves.

Readings

Pause at this moment and complete the following readings. They offer some insight into what it is like to grow old.

When does someone attain old age?

http://ohioline.osu.edu/ss-fact/0101.html

Sociological theories on ageing

http://allnurses-breakroom.com/geriatrics-aging-elderly/theories-aging-part-412760.html

Reflection

Considering the data from the readings and how the panellists responded to the questions, it is clear that becoming older is not just a physiological degenerative response. Anne says that ageing is do with 'your situation and your background and your upbringing'. Theo speaks about 'the ability to contribute to society or to sustain oneself'. How do these responses now align with what you believe ageing is about?

Inquiry

There are many ways in which we can define ageing. Although it is a biological response, it is also about how we live our lives and see ourselves. Ageing has both an emotional and a sociological perspective. It is holistic and not just linear within a biological framework. We also see ageing and the older person within the framework of our own experiences and our personal and cultural values.

Action

A Consider the ageing process and how the panellists view what it is to be old. How do the different viewpoints (theories) of ageing affect your practice?

B How do we stereotype our older clients when we provide healthcare services? Do we stereotype our clients by assuming how they feel about their personal ageing experiences? How can your organisations better manage these stereotypes?

C When developing organisational policies, how do you contextualise policy that considers an individual's perception of ageing? Is it possible to do this? Is it possible to completely remove ageist attitudes from the workplace?

Readings

Read the following articles and view the video clip and consider how they fit with what the panellists say.

New Zealand's oldest driver: 'I do not feel old'

www.youtube.com/watch?v=PlJQYEbHvxo

Reflection

Now reflect on what you have learned from the chapter so far.

1. Do we prescribe to preset ideas about what it is to be old and plan our care accordingly?

2. Do we consider generational differences of the older person? Or do we currently offer a 'one-size-fits-all' service? Does a 75 year old have the same ideas about ageing as a 95 year old? Do they need the same type of aged care service?

3. As the baby boomers are now ageing and moving into what could be considered 'old', how are we planning to contextualise provision of aged care to support their needs? Do we need to change aged care practices for this generation?

A FINAL WORD

Although there appears to be some consensus that to be deemed old you should be over 60 years of age, there is no real and definitive number given. If you are of Aboriginal and/or Torres Strait Islander descent, that figure changes to over 50 years of age. Even when we consider the individual and ask them what age is old, the number varies. Using the government's rulings on set aged care entitlements does not realistically determine what age is old. These determinants are influenced by an increasing number of social, demographic and economic factors. With no numerical definition of what is old, we must realistically define what it is to be old by other means. However, for those of us who work within, and for, the aged care communities we need to ensure that we do not exclude people from care due to a numerical value. We also do not want to presume that a person who falls within a certain numerical value age-wise requires specific aged care requirements.

This section has briefly touched on perceptions of ageing. From listening to our panellists and undertaking some of the readings, we can conclude that ageing is not just a biological process. Ageing is a holistic process that is about the person: who they are, what they feel and what their experiences are. It is difficult to define who is an older person unless we consider all these factors. Offering a one-size-fits-all service to all people who are deemed to be old would fail to consider people's unique differences.

By now you should better understand perceptions of not only what is old, but also what it is to age. Ageing starts at whatever time an individual believes it to be for them. The older person's needs are also highly individual. As one of the panellists remarked after the videoing, 'If I ever have to be put into a nursing home, they had better have plenty of Bob Marley and heavy rock for me to listen to plus some play stations to use. If I have to watch afternoon TV, play bingo or listen to soothing music I will go mad!'

CHAPTER 2

Positive Ageing

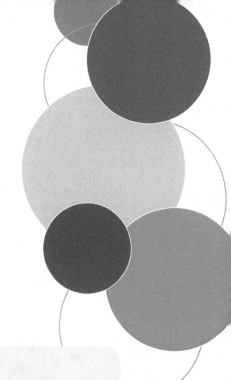

INTRODUCTION

This chapter introduces you to the concept of positive ageing. There are two discrete sections to this chapter, each focusing on lifestyle and social connectedness. The chapter contains stories from people living their lives actively within the community in their quest to maintain health through the positive aspect of ageing.

The first story incorporates five women who are members of a women's social networking group. These women discuss the importance of socialising, making new friends and having fun as they 'grow up'.

The second story is told by Ron and Larry, two men aged 80 and 84 years respectively. They discuss the importance of maintaining a positive and fulfilling lifestyle following their retirement, and how they do this by integrating their hobbies, family and the learning of new skills.

Before you begin the Red Hat Ladies' story ... How perceptions of positive ageing shape practice

At some time through your coursework you may have considered: 'how old is too old?' Once again, it is time to reflect on this question. If society is ageing and everyone is to continue to be an active member of the community for longer, at what age should one be expected to stop learning, growing and having fun? Consider the following questions. You may wish to discuss these with your colleagues to gauge their opinions too. It might surprise you what you find!

- What do you think a person over the age of 65 years does for fun?

- Would you do the same thing for fun?

- Could you tell a person over the age of 85 years a risqué joke? Do you think that they would understand the meaning? If not, why not?

- Would you join a group that expects you to dress up in costume when you go out to social events (i.e. restaurants, coffee shops etc.)?

- Now, what would you think if a group of aged persons over 70 years dressed up in costumes and came to that same restaurant while you were sitting at the next table with your friends?

Understanding how perspectives change is an important aspect of learning more about the wants and needs of the community as they age. Lifestyle choices play a key role in determining how individuals will successfully meet their advancing years, and contributes to the health and wellbeing of the individual. Maintaining active friendships throughout life underpin the social fabric of society. Most individuals thrive on day-to-day interactions with others. The relationships that are built through this exchange can play a key role in the quality of life for the aged person. While there are many social groups that one might join, finding the 'right fit' is often difficult for many individuals.

Some older persons are fearful of joining new groups because they are unfamiliar with what is expected of them, or what commitment or expenses are needed. Those who do take up the opportunity to join groups, clubs or societies strive to continue to learn and participate in social activities within the community that promote a sense of wellbeing and positivity within their lives.

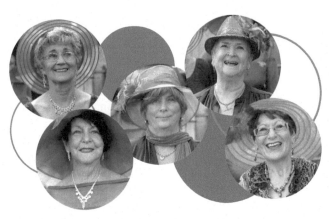

The Red Hat Ladies' story

 Begin viewing the Red Hat Ladies' story to the start of 'Bubbles and butterflies—learning to have fun!' or read the transcript.

Reflection

Consider the different reasons each one gives for joining the group. You may have noticed some common themes in the comments made and also some differences. You will also have noticed the attire (or dress) that each of the ladies is wearing and the differing ages within the group.

1. Identify the common themes that have brought the women together to be part of this group.

2. Explain why some of the group may have chosen a specific nickname as part of the group. Is this significant?

3. Discuss the comment made by one member of the group in relation to joining a group that is for 'fun', as women usually have many responsibilities in their life.

4. The ladies laugh over the use of the term 'growing up' rather than growing older. What do you think might be the significance of them using this term?

Bubbles and butterflies—learning to have fun!

The Red Hat Ladies go on to discuss how the group has helped them grow and cope with issues that may be occurring in their personal lives. They use the camaraderie and fun of the group as a mechanism for working through these problems. Dawn comments on the joy that each member brings to the group. As you continue watching the video, see what fun the ladies have learning to enjoy each other's company.

 Continue viewing the Red Hat Ladies' story to 'Outings, friendships and fun' or read the transcript.

Inquiry

In their story, the Red Hat Ladies go on to discuss the importance of learning skills and developing self-confidence as part of this journey. Extending themselves in this fun role enables them to maintain friendships and social networking that may have been lost if not for these groups. 'Making the most of every day' is highlighted as an aspect of this as the members take time to be happy.

Giles et al. (2005) conducted a longitudinal study of 1477 Australians over 70 years of age in both community and residential facilities over a 10-year period. During this time, it was found that having a strong link with social networks enhanced the older individual's lifestyle. These authors also found that friendships and family interactions facilitated increased health and wellbeing and promoted optimal survival rates over the study period. You may like to take the time to read this interesting research for yourself.

Giles LC, Glonek GFV, Luszcz MA & Andrews GR 2005 Effect of social networks on 10 year survival in very old Australians: the Australian longitudinal study of aging. Journal of Epidemiology and Community Health 59(7):574–579

http://jech.bmj.com/content/59/7/574.short

There is a range of research into social isolation and ageing. Only two have been chosen here to highlight the impact that friendships and participation in networking or lifestyle activities might have on the individual.

The second study is by Steptoe et al. (2013) who carried out a longitudinal study to consider social isolation and the experience of loneliness within the ageing population, and how this might impact on the mortality rate. While loneliness was not independent of the health issues or other contributing demographic factors, both social isolation and loneliness was found to contribute to a reduced quality of life and wellbeing. You may wish to also review this study as part of your work.

Steptoe A, Shankar A, Demakakos P, Wardle J 2013 Social isolation, loneliness, and all-cause mortality in older men and women. Proceedings of National Academy of Science 110(15):5797–5801

www.pnas.org/content/110/15/5797

Outings, friendships and fun

There are a range of clubs and groups that individuals may join as they get older. Volunteering is also an activity that many individuals take up in their later years. The Red Hat Ladies go on to discuss why they enjoy being part of the group.

 Finish viewing the Red Hat Ladies' story or read the transcript.

Reflection

1. Consider why the Ladies enjoy being part of the group.
2. Why is it important to 'put their make-up on and dress up'?
3. Why might it be important that Sandy is able to have a shared relationship with others and 'leave everything else behind'?
4. What do you think Carol means when she says 'it's all about the girls' and that women are responsible for many things?
5. What is the difference between a volunteering group and a social networking group? Why

might ageing individuals choose one over the other?
6. How important is it for ageing individuals to continue to 'push their boundaries'?

Last word—beauty through photography

Lastly, a reference text has been added merely for your own pleasure. *Advanced Style* by Ari Seth Cohen (2012) is a wonderful find and a lovely addition to any collection as a coffee table book. It depicts the pure elegance of the ageing female, fashionably through photography. The book celebrates the over-60s female enjoying their life with confidence and flair.

Before you begin Ron and Larry's story ... How perceptions of positive ageing shape practice

The story from the Red Hat Ladies gave you an opportunity to develop an understanding of the women's view of participating in group activities. The second video tells the story of two men who are also part of a social group. Before commencing their story, it is important to gauge your perceptions (and maybe those of your colleagues) in relation to the difference between these two gender groups as they age. Take the time to reflect on the following.

• Are there differences between how and what attracts men and women to join social groups?

• What do you think each gender group hopes to gain from the interaction? Do you think this is different?

• Do these goals change as the person ages?

• Consider the impact that professional, financial or health status might have on the older individual's choice to join or participate in a social group. What are the key drivers and choices that the person will make related to these issues?

• Do you believe that people over the age of 70 can learn the same skills as younger people? If not, why not?

• Do you believe that people over the age of 70 find it more difficult than younger people to learn to use a computer? If not, why not?

- Imagine that you are setting up a healthy lifestyle group for an ageing community within a designated area in your local community. What type of information would you need to know? (You may wish to discuss this with your colleagues and use it as a project in your future practice.)

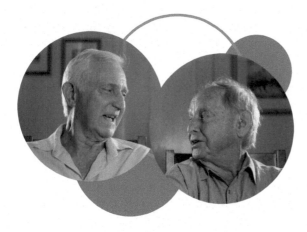

Ron and Larry's story

 Begin viewing Ron and Larry's story to 'Keeping busy in retirement' or read the transcript.

Reflection

Both Ron and Larry discuss their involvement in the Wooden Boat Association, as well as their other hobbies. Larry goes on to talk about the particular tasks he has taken up since he retired. Many of these are now consuming more of his time than when he was working.

1. Why is it important to have a hobby once you retire?

2. How does the group that Ron and Larry are in differ from the Red Hat Ladies?

3. Larry comments on maintaining contact with past acquaintances and mentions that he writes the newsletter and also undertakes other computer tasks.

   a. How important is it to keep in touch with past contacts as a person ages?

   b. What percentage of the ageing community are computer literate?

   c. How important is it for the ageing population to have access to the internet and the wider community via a computer?

Inquiry

Moving into retirement may often result in considerable changes for the individual. The obvious one relates to financial status and links with friends or work colleagues. However, the key aspects in ensuring that this transition is smooth and easier to manage are developing new relationships, learning new skills and taking up long-forgotten or new hobbies. Sharing skills may significantly improve the quality of life for the ageing person. As a future healthcare professional, you can enable individuals to maintain their lifestyle and independence through socialisation and community connectedness. Consider how you might assist in this.

McLaughlin et al. (2010) conducted a study which reviewed the impact of gender-specific social support associated with mortality and morbidity rates in later life. They found that women have increased social networks, while men's health was impacted by reduced social support structures. Overall satisfaction was seen where there was reduced support across both genders. This study highlights the importance of ensuring that structures are in place throughout the lifespan to support the individual and provide a broad spectrum of interaction with the wider community physically, psychologically, emotionally and spiritually.

Take the time to read McLaughlin et al.'s (2010) article.

McLaughlin D, Vagenas D, Pachana NA, Begum N, Dobson A 2010 Gender differences in social network size and satisfaction in adults in their 70s. Journal of Health Psychology 15(5):671–679
www.ncbi.nlm.nih.gov/pubmed/20603290

Financial planning and failing to plan

One of the key responses to health and wellbeing for the ageing individual post-retirement is the ability to plan for this stage in the individual's life. Lack of financial support prior to, and after, retirement may pose a detrimental effect on the physical, psychological and emotional wellbeing of the individual. It is therefore imperative that financial planning play a role in care discussions between healthcare professionals and their clients or residents. The changing face of healthcare is such that registered nurses are more often thrust into the role of case manager for the client, providing a raft of resources and support including not only the physical aspects of their care but also the psychological and environmental support structures required to sustain an individual throughout their life.

In their story, both Ron and Larry discuss their financial planning and how this differed, based on their preparedness for retirement. Take the time to reflect on these differences.

 Continue viewing Ron and Larry's story to 'Developing computer skills' or read the transcript.

Reflection

Consider the differences between Ron's planning for retirement and Larry's lack of financial planning or, as Larry states, 'failure to plan'. While some of this was not of his making, there are significant repercussions when one is not able to successfully meet future living and healthcare expenses.

Reflect on the following questions. You might like to discuss these with your colleagues.

1. What impact might there be if one fails to financially plan for retirement?

2. How might you as a future healthcare professional support an ageing client or resident who is struggling with the intricacies of financial planning?

3. What skills might the older person require to support them into the future if they are to manage effectively in this environment?

Learning computing and new skills

One area challenging the ageing community has been the advent of computers and the internet. Mobile phones and electronic banking may also pose significant difficulties for the older person. However, many have taken up the challenge like Ron and Larry learning new skills. Ron comments on this 'technology time warp' as he explains the purchase of a new phone. While advances in technology are moving at a fast pace, it is important to remember that the ageing person still needs assistance to understand this new world. Many are embracing these changes but some may not find this so easy. Ron provides

anecdotal evidence of this. Watch the rest of their story to see how they manage with technology.

 Finish viewing Ron and Larry's story or read the transcript.

Life doesn't stop when you retire

As Ron says, 'there's still an awful lot to do!' So what are we waiting for? As healthcare professionals, it is imperative that we have a clear understanding of the ageing person's vision of how they want to continue to live their life, where they are headed and how we can assist them to make this happen. This is not an easy task, based on the physical, emotional and financial hardships that often face the ageing community. However, with the added clinical knowledge, skill and respect for clients or residents, healthcare providers will be able to effectively support and advocate for them.

The Further readings and references for this chapter at the end of the book contain examples of some of the clubs/networks available to individuals wishing to become a member of a group within their own community. This list provides only a brief example of what is available.

Action

A Describe what is meant by positive ageing. Is it more than just maintaining one's own physical health? What are the aspects that might impact on positive ageing?

B After viewing the two videos, what gender differences do you identify in building social networks? Using a primary healthcare focus, how does your healthcare role include the promotion of a healthy and positive lifestyle within the ageing population? How has the use of technology assisted the older person in developing social networks?

C Consider the current government policies encouraging older people to be more proactive in their choice of healthcare. How will this change the Australian healthcare system in the future? Review current social theories of ageing and critically reflect upon these to consider how valid they are for current and future generations of older people. Compare these to the discussions within the videos.

A FINAL WORD

The concept of positive ageing is not just living longer but having a quality of life where the individual may experience choice and satisfaction with his or her own achievements. It is important that these choices are grounded not just in the physical wellbeing but also in the psychological, emotional and spiritual health of the person. Enabling this through social connectedness and empowerment is an important aspect of the healthcare professional's role, allowing them to facilitate an improved quality of life for the individual.

This chapter has provided a brief insight into a number of individual stories within two videos. These are only a brief glimpse into the many stories that exist within the community where older Australians are making a significant contribution to everyday life.

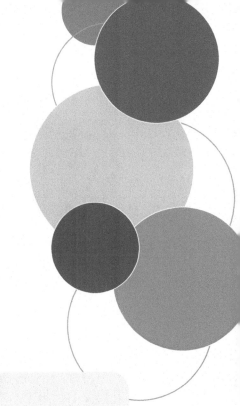

CHAPTER 3

The Indigenous Older Person

INTRODUCTION

This chapter consists of two stories that provide distinct perspectives of the concept of ageing as an indigenous person, particularly in Australia and the Torres Strait Islands. Each story has key areas of interest that draw on the experience of the individual within a contemporary Australian context and considers the issues that may impact on the consumer, the community and the healthcare professional within this environment.

Odette Best identifies herself as an Indigenous registered nurse who has lived among five generations of her Indigenous family. She explores the concept of healthy ageing for Indigenous community members from both personal experience and as a health professional.

Ali Drummond is an Indigenous member of the Torres Strait Islands community. Ali discusses his family's experience living in a Torres Strait community that has a large multicultural history. He also shares his personal experience caring for elders and ageing people from the Torres Strait Islands, both in the community and within an aged care facility.

Before you begin ... How history of a culture can shape current practice

Think about your knowledge of the indigenous community of your own country. What do you know of their history? How do you think they were affected when the country was resettled or 'colonised' into its current form of government and legislations?

1. What do you think it must be like to live within a family community that has been taken over by new laws and rulers that don't understand the beliefs of your family or community?

2. How might this shape your personal or family values, lifestyle, choices and opportunities within the modern day running of the country?

3. Are you aware of any differences between people who are referred to as Aboriginal Australians and Torres Strait Islanders? How would you find out?

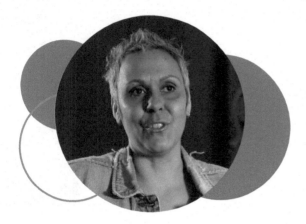

historical, contemporary, social and cultural factors on individual health outcomes. It is essential to listen to the experiences of Indigenous Australians as many of them have experienced first-hand the complex factors that have influenced health in general both within their community and within their own family. Understanding their experiences assists the health professional to also understand their health beliefs, which ultimately reflect their attitudes, fears and values about health and the assistance provided from the healthcare system.

Odette's story

 Continue viewing Odette's story to 'Access to health services' or read the transcript.

 Begin viewing Odette's story to 'Historical perspective and repercussions on health' or read the transcript.

Reflection

Odette discusses the history of Indigenous Australians and mentions that government officials continued to remove children from their family up to the mid-1970s.

1. Think about the years your parents and grandparents were born. How would your family be different if they had experienced similar 'interventions' from government bodies? How do you think their attitudes to you participating in the health industry would be different to their attitudes now?

2. It has been demonstrated that lifestyle factors contribute significantly to disease, particularly cardiovascular disease and diabetes (two major diseases in the Indigenous population). How do you think the introduction of the typical Australian diet affected the Indigenous population who until then had lived off naturally occurring 'clean' foods such as fish and other food collected from nature?

3. Consider the factors that may impact on an Indigenous Australian's ability to assimilate within the Australian community. How will these factors be overcome (in the short or long term)?

You may wish to review the following website that is a helpful resource regarding health issues of Indigenous people in Australia.

Australian Indigenous Health InfoNet, Overview of Australian Indigenous health status 2012

www.healthinfonet.ecu.edu.au/health-facts/overviews

Reflection

1. List the challenges identified by Odette.

2. Can you think of any more to add to the list that she has not identified? If so, add them now.

3. Odette states that 'for many Aboriginal communities across Australia eldership is revered so we don't, where we can, separate our elders and our community from the generations that are actually running behind them'. How do your views about the elderly in your community compare?

Inquiry

Indigenous people across the world and in Australia often have poorer health than non-Indigenous people. This situation is reflected in the health status of Aboriginal and Torres Strait Islander peoples who die much younger than the rest of the Australian population. The Australian Bureau of Statistics reports that life expectancy for Aboriginal and Torres Strait Islander males and females was 11.5 and 9.7 years shorter than other Australian males and females (Australian Bureau of Statistics, 2009).

Reasons for the poorer health status of Aboriginal and Torres Strait Islander peoples are complex and non-Indigenous Australians can best appreciate this by considering the impact of significant

Accessing health services

Encouraging people to access health services when they need them is essential to promote positive ageing. It is therefore imperative that people within the community trust and feel comfortable accessing services.

 Finish viewing Odette's story or read the transcript.

Reflection

1. Do you think the distrust in the Indigenous community is justified?
2. What impacts could this have on the health of ageing Indigenous Australians?
3. What issues may arise for clients that come from an Aboriginal background, who are then diagnosed with an illness such as cardiovascular disease?
4. How might you as a health professional assist?

Inquiry

The National Aboriginal Community Controlled Health Organisation (NACCHO) was established to recognise the importance of trust building and empowerment. It aims to inform Indigenous Australians about health issues and services as well as promote access and equity for the community.

In 2013, the *NACCHO 10 Point Plan* for assisting Aboriginals to maintain a healthy lifestyle was published. It can be downloaded for free from www.naccho.org.au/. Access the plan and consider the following questions.

1. How can this plan be implemented?
2. What potential barriers can you see?
3. What suggestions do you have to overcome the potential barriers?

Action

A Describe how important it is to be aware of a community's history. How might you ensure that you translate this awareness into your day-to-day healthcare practice?

B Review your reflections above and relate this to the aged care/clinical setting in which you are either currently employed or have attended on clinical placement. How would this current setting provide sensitivity to the issues previously faced by an Indigenous resident through organisational policies and procedures? Why?

C Critically review current literature in relation to managing Indigenous clients/residents within an ageing population that reflects cultural sensitivity. Consider how well this literature informs current practice.

Review your organisational policies and procedures in relation to potential barriers that could create difficulty in providing appropriate care to an Aboriginal elder. Highlight and document the changes required to ensure that it is consistent with acknowledgment of specific needs for Aboriginal elders.

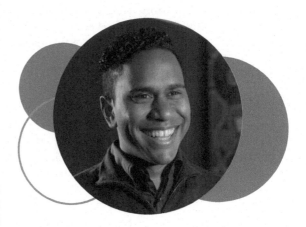

Ali's story

 View Ali's story or read the transcript.

Reflection

As mentioned in the introduction, Ali is a Torres Strait Islander. He talks about his own experiences with ageing, particularly within the Torres Strait Islander community. His experiences are both personal and professional, coming from within his own family and his work in an aged care facility.

1. What did Ali consider the most important aspects when caring for an older Torres Strait Islander?
2. How do you think that fits with current concepts of workloads within an aged care facility?
3. How can any potential problems be overcome to ensure appropriate care is provided?

13

Inquiry

Because of the earlier mortality age for Aboriginal and Torres Strait Islander peoples, old age is considered by both the government and the Aboriginal communities to start at 50 years of age (Dance et al., 2004).

If you have not already done so, view this section of the video or read through the transcript for discussion of community members ignoring medical conditions due to the widespread acceptance within the community that they will experience these conditions.

Accessing health services

As mentioned in Ali's story, community members accept chronic disease in their life, even before they are 40 years of age. This acceptance means that there is little motivation, if any, to seek assistance in the prevention or treatment of chronic disease.

Reflection

1. How do you react if someone tells you that what you do may be negatively impacting on your health; for example, lack of physical exercise, sleep patterns, not enough water intake and so on?

2. How do you choose what healthy interventions you undertake?

3. How important is it to have a sense of self-empowerment? How might a health professional support this notion for the individual?

4. How would you assist in health promotion activities in a Torres Strait Islander community?

Action

A Describe the importance of family and community networks in the care of the ageing person within an Aboriginal or Torres Strait Islander environment.

B Explore the concept of family involvement in holistic care. What is your future role in promoting community and family involvement in the care of an Indigenous elder?

C Consider the currently promoted identity of a typical Australian in television or print media. How does this reflect the identity of an Aboriginal or Torres Strait Islander? Identify how this impacts on the health of an Aboriginal or Torres Strait Islander. Identify organisations and potential policies that may assist in promoting healthy ageing within the Indigenous Australian community.

A FINAL WORD

As a healthcare professional, it is essential to have a broad understanding of the complexities of the often differing needs of Australia's Indigenous population. As this population ages, it is important not to stereotype your views of the needs of these groups. However, you must understand how Indigenous experiences within Australia can affect your efforts to show understanding and establish trust and rapport. Remember that the client or family you care for is the best source of information about individual cultural needs.

CHAPTER 4

Ageing Within a Culturally Diverse Society

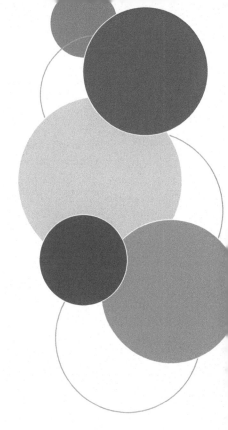

INTRODUCTION

The two stories within this chapter examine ageing within a multicultural setting. Each story has key areas of interest that draw on the experience of the individual within a contemporary Australian context and considers the issues that may impact on the consumer, the community and the healthcare professional within this environment.

Mercedes Sepulveda is a health professional who will explore cultural diversity in a broad context, providing an overview of what it is to live and age within a culturally diverse community. Mercedes is of Chilean descent and has extensive experience working with a range of cultural groups within the ageing community.

Rafael Pacheco is an ageing El Salvadorian refugee from a culturally diverse background, whose second language is English. Rafael discusses his family's experience integrating with the Australian culture, the highs and lows of learning new ways within a different culture and factors affecting their transition to this change.

Before you begin ... How perceptions about culture shape practice

Consider what you know about your community and the people that live in your neighbourhood. Think about your family history and also that of your friends. Before viewing the stories (or reading the transcripts) in this chapter, reflect on the questions below and consider your views about diversity within your community. Also reflect on the needs of the community and how there are met each day.

1. What do you know of your family history? Are you a first-generation Australian? If not, what is your heritage?

2. Consider what it must be like for an older person living within a cultural environment other than their birth one. How does this differ from your own cultural experience?

3. How might this shape your personal or family values, lifestyle, choices and opportunities?

4. What is the demographic spread of cultural groups within your local community, and why is this the case? In there any reason that specific

cultural groups choose to reside together in one area?

5. What services or resources are you currently familiar with that would be available or useful to support an ageing population within the Australian multicultural community?

Ageing versus ageism

Understanding the difference between the terms 'ageing' and 'ageism' is very important when considering the concept of multiculturalism. Reflect on your understanding of the difference between these two terms. Do you know what the difference is? Many definitions may be found on the internet or via library resources. What is the impact of ageism on the current ageing population? You might like to reflect on the definitions for each term and how the concept of ageism affects the ageing society and those who interact with them. Take the time to review this topic for yourself and document your findings so that you may refer to this later.

In the first story, Mercedes discusses ageing and ageism within the context of the Australian culture and the impact on individuals who may be settling within this country. She goes on to discuss the challenges for the individual and how Australian society may address this through community action. This introductory discussion provides a basis for healthcare professionals to develop a better understanding of the barriers that influence those consumers ageing within an Australian multicultural environment.

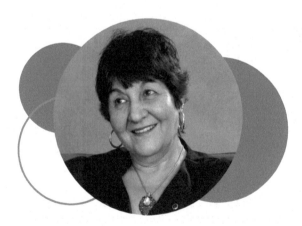

Mercedes' story

 Begin viewing Mercedes' story to 'We need to look at diversity' or read the transcript.

Reflection

Consider what you have learned so far. You may also wish to review your understanding of the challenges to cultural diversity within an Australian context. Take the time to identify the various cultural groups within your local community and how these differ in terms of their healthcare needs and the challenges that impact on each.

1. List the challenges identified by Mercedes in her story.

2. Can you think of any more to add to the list that she has not identified? If so, add them now.

3. What are your thoughts when someone says to you that healthcare for the multicultural community in Australia should be 'one size fits all'?

Inquiry

The Australian Population and Migration Research Centre (APMRC) at the University of Adelaide's School of Social Sciences supports the multicultural environment. It does this through the storage and dissemination of specialised information in the areas of health and aged care, population projections, demographical and spatial analysis as well as multicultural modelling and web-based set up. A diverse range of information is available at their website identifying demographic and targeted data in relation to specific needs groups across the spectrum of the Australian population. At this point you might like to access the website and search for your area to identify its specific needs groups.

Australian Population and Migration Research Centre (APMRC)

www.adelaide.edu.au/apmrc

 Continue viewing Mercedes' story to 'Accessing services' or read the transcript.

Reflection

Mercedes discusses the issues related to settling in a new country, adaptation and how to manage this change. Mercedes goes on to identify the status of migrants and new settlers as 'offshore refugees' or 'onshore asylum seekers'. You might like to research the terms to become more familiar with these.

1. What is the difference between these two terms?

2. How will this refugee or asylum seeker status impact on the individual's 'standing' within the community and their ability to access healthcare?

3. How will these issues be further exacerbated if the person is an ageing refugee?

4. What avenues (healthcare agencies) are available to meet the needs of both groups?

5. Consider the factors that may impact on the individual's ability to assimilate within the Australian community. How will these factors be overcome (in the short or long term)?

Accessing services

Equipping the healthcare professional with the appropriate knowledge, skills and training to support the individual within the multicultural environment is vital to ensuring a healthy ageing experience. It is therefore imperative that staff have the appropriate attitude and ability to work with this diverse cultural group, free from bias and discrimination. It is crucial that resources such as adequate translation services are available in order to provide optimal healthcare. Mercedes discusses the case of a consumer that experienced a poor response to a culturally sensitive issue when receiving healthcare.

 Continue viewing Mercedes' story to 'Cultural sensitivity' or read the transcript.

You may also wish to review the Alzheimer's Australia website for the National Cross Cultural Dementia Network (NCCDN). This advisory body advocates on behalf of Alzheimer's Australia on a wide range of issues in relation to culturally diverse communities and consumers experiencing dementia. The NCCDN has a number of mandated objectives.

National Cross Cultural Dementia Network

www.fightdementia.org.au/understanding-dementia/cultural-diversity.aspx

Reflection

1. Have you experienced any instances where clients or residents have been provided with treatment that is contrary to their cultural beliefs? What was the result?

2. Can you list any examples of cultural stereotyping that occurs on a daily basis?

3. Are these stereotypical examples used by others or by yourself? How have these come about within the community?

4. Have you or your colleagues experienced or seen any examples of racism/discrimination within the workplace or elsewhere? If so, can you provide an example and the outcome?

5. What issues may arise for clients from a multicultural background who are diagnosed with an illness such as dementia?

6. How might this impact not only on the client or resident, but also on the family and their community?

Inquiry

Healthcare professionals should be supported in caring for culturally diverse clients and residents through the development of a multicultural practice framework (MPF). Client-focused service provision is inherent in this model that seeks to value the experience of the individual and enable staff to deliver services within a culturally sensitive and supportive context. View the rest of Mercedes' story for information on MPFs or read her transcript.

 Finish viewing Mercedes' story or read the transcript.

Action

A Describe how important it is to be culturally sensitive to the needs of your clients and residents who you care for within the community or residential setting. How might you ensure that you enact or display this sensitivity in your day-to-day care practice?

B Review your current understanding of the MPF discussed. Relate this to the aged care or clinical setting in which you are either currently employed or have attended on clinical placement. How does this current setting provide evidence of this framework through organisational policies and procedures? How well do you believe this framework is implemented in the care of the elderly client? Outline your rationale.

C Critically review current literature on cultural diversity and managing culturally and linguistically diverse (CALD) clients and residents within an ageing population. Consider how well this literature informs current practice.

Review your organisational policies and procedures in relation to current aged care reforms. Identify any alignment or misalignment between reform and current policy. Highlight and document the changes needed in your organisation's document to make it consistent with current legislation.

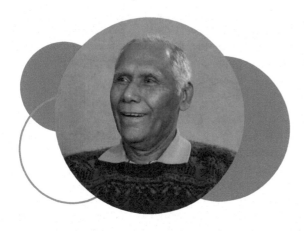

Rafael's story

 Begin viewing Rafael's story to 'Language barriers and jobs' or read the transcript.

As mentioned in the introduction, the second story is an interview with Rafael Pacheco, an ageing man from El Salvador. Rafael travelled with his family from Costa Rica to Australia as a refugee. They were placed in a migrant hostel in Melbourne for the first 12 months prior to relocating to Brisbane.

He talks about his experiences settling in a new country, learning the language, receiving residency status and understanding the culture, as well as his rights within this new setting. Rafael has identified a number of challenges from his experience and the services that the migrant hostel offered to support him and his family through this process.

Reflection

1. How many migrant hostels exist across Australia at present and how are these funded?
2. What services are offered by migrant hostels within Australia today?

3. What are some of the concerns that refugees might have when entering this type of facility?
4. How would you react if you were displaced from everything and everyone familiar and relocated to a migrant facility?
5. What would make this experience more tenable?

Inquiry

Distance, isolation, size of cultural community, language barrier and cultural shift are all key drivers in making settlement either a positive or a negative experience for the migrant. Rafael goes on to explain the difficulties older migrants face in adjusting to the changes of moving to a new country, learning a new language and adjusting to new ways of living. He states the importance of a number of factors as impacting on the individual's experience including age, expectation and level of education.

Language barriers and jobs

Rafael discusses working as a professional and how his experience differed from that of others.

 Continue viewing Rafael's story to 'Raising children and grandchildren' or read the transcript.

You may also like to now peruse one of the readings listed at the end of this book. The briefing paper listed below provides an overview of the healthcare professional working with older people from a CALD background. This literature facilitates understanding of the management of CALD clients within the community in response to issues of isolation, vulnerability and challenges experienced from loss of homeland.

Social Policy Research Centre and The Benevolent Society October 2010 Supporting older people from culturally diverse backgrounds. Research to Practice Briefing 4. The Benevolent Society. https://www.sprc.unsw.edu.au/media/SPRCFile/10_Report_BenSoc_ResearchtoPractice4.pdf

Rafael goes on to discuss being a grandparent in later life and the issues that arise from raising children in a different culture and another language. He also talks about changes to living conditions, a person's environment, his self-image and his self-esteem.

Continue viewing Rafael's story to 'Settling in and frustrations' or read the transcript.

Reflection

Many of the concerns that migrants and culturally diverse individuals within an ageing population have are not so different from yourself. Take the time to reflect on your own life and new experiences as they occur such as finding a new job, learning new skills, meeting new people and so on.

1. What factors might affect your ability to manage new situations such as those mentioned above?

2. What would make these new situations a more positive experience for you, both emotionally and practically?

3. How important is it to have a strong sense of self or a positive self-esteem? How might a health professional support this notion for the individual?

4. Think about a situation you have been in where you have not known anyone. How did you feel? What did you do?

5. Have you ever been in a situation where you did not know or understand the language? How did you feel? What did you do?

6. What did you learn from the experience?

Settling in and frustrations

These situations are very real for the individual who is displaced or has relocated to a new country. It is imperative that healthcare professionals have a clear understanding of the needs of the person, especially as they age. Elderly individuals will be vulnerable through their inability to grasp the language nuances and cultural differences, and may become more prone to isolation. Often those who come from a professional background find it difficult to assimilate into a new culture at their previous level and become emotionally traumatised.

Rafael provides an example of this in his video and reiterates the importance of positive self-esteem and adequate services to support culturally and linguistically diverse people.

 Continue viewing Rafael's story to 'Accessing social services' or read the transcript.

Accessing social services

As mentioned in Mercedes' story, it is important that healthcare professionals are familiar with the needs of culturally diverse clients who may or may not be new to the community. Access to information is paramount for the individual, including knowing where services are and how to access them. As Rafael discusses, individuals from multicultural backgrounds feel safest within their own houses and may become isolated as they grow older if they are not provided with appropriate healthcare information and resources.

Healthcare professionals must embrace different cultural experiences and empower individuals to access healthcare through information sharing, interpreter services, drop-in facilities and community access points. As previously mentioned, having appropriate resources is central to delivering healthcare services effectively. Using the skills and networks within multicultural communities will assist in facilitating positive health outcomes for the ageing community.

View the rest of Rafael's video for his experience as a community worker or read the transcript. Rafael goes on to highlight the difficulties encountered by the multicultural community when accessing services and the inappropriate use of children as interpreters. Lack of sensitivity to the needs of individuals and their family can lead to frustration, isolation and frayed tempers.

 Finish viewing Rafael's story or read the transcript.

You may also read the following article that explores the concept of how older Australians from diverse cultural backgrounds contribute to community through grandparenting, maintaining and promoting their culture and as a cultural advisor to their communities.

Warburton J, McLaughlin D 2007 Passing on our culture: how older Australians from diverse cultural backgrounds contribute to civil society. Journal of Cross-Cultural Gerontology 22(1):47–60

http://link.springer.com/article/10.1007/s10823-006-9012-4

Reflection

Whether you are a beginner or an experienced health professional, there are a diverse range of considerations to be made when either planning for or

19

implementing care of a person from a multicultural background, never more so as this person ages. Reflect on what these challenges might be.

1. What are the key drivers in relation to providing healthcare services for the CALD client?

2. What are the challenges for the CALD client as he or she gets older?

3. How will the healthcare services meet that challenge?

4. What practical strategies can you use in your day-to-day practice to make the person and his or her family more comfortable with the care you wish to deliver?

Action

A Describe the importance of family and community networks in caring for an ageing person within a multicultural environment.

B Explore the concepts of 'quality of life' and 'quality of time' as identified by Rafael at the end of the video as a reason for continuing to move forward. What is your future role in ensuring that these concepts underpin the care for the CALD client within the healthcare setting?

C Consider the current and often controversial Australian debate on migration policy. Critically analyse the government's policy to determine the management of the diverse healthcare needs for the older migrant population. Identify any gaps in service provision, the resources needed to fill these gaps and how these might be overcome into the future knowing what you do now about the best approach to self-management, support and challenges for CALD clients.

A FINAL WORD

Australia's population is culturally and linguistically diverse and so caring for often differing needs can be complex. It is important that you do not stereotype your views of this group's needs as the population ages. There are also significant differences within specific cultural groups that must be considered. The cultural safety of both your client and yourself must be considered at all times.

The development of a multicultural practice framework is imperative as a foundation for providing healthcare services that meet the individual and family needs of diverse communities. The stories of both Mercedes and Rafael have provided a brief snapshot of their experiences and understanding of multiculturalism.

CHAPTER 5

Sexuality in the Later Years

INTRODUCTION

This chapter looks at the concept of sexuality and the older person. As part of this chapter, Dr Cindy Jones introduces you to sexuality as a broad multi-dimensional construct, outlining the many facets of sexuality as we all age. This includes a person's need to share in a relationship with others through sexual expression that may involve not only the physical act of sex but also an individual's need to share the experience of intimacy, companionship or friendship with another person, or the need to find romance and love in any form and sexual orientation.

There is a range of literature available on this topic, both paper- and web-based. Some have been added to the Further readings and references for this chapter at the end of the book. Dr Jones' story also offers insight into contemporary issues in relation to sexuality and ageing for clients and residents within the community or residential environment. This provides you with the opportunity to reflect on your own knowledge, opinions and cultural or family values that may have developed over time in relation to this topic, as she goes on to discuss the concept of sexuality through the eyes of the older person.

Before you begin ... How perceptions of sexuality as we age shape practice

Think about your own views and how these have shaped your perceptions over time. Also consider how the views and opinions of others may be similar or different to your own, and the impact of these on outcomes for clients. Before going on to view Dr Cindy's story (or read the transcript) take the time to reflect on and answer the questions below.

1. Consider your personal views on sexuality. How have your views on sexuality been shaped over time?

2. To what extent have these views been impacted on by your personal values and your background or family life?

3. Have these views or opinions changed over time or are they the same as when you were younger (growing up)? If not, what has happened to change your point of view and why?

4. How might your views and the opinions of others shape healthcare practice and organisational decisions when caring for clients or residents?

Community perceptions of sexuality

Notions of sexuality are constantly evolving in line with community expectations and values. Health professionals need to keep abreast of education and training opportunities to ensure that they are up to date with the changing needs of the ageing population. We have all grown up with different perceptions of sexuality and what this means. In addition, each person has a view on how old someone should be to have sex and when this should stop. This is a perspective of sexuality and ageing that may have a positive or detrimental impact on the care and support given to an individual within the community or a residential facility. How the health professional responds to clients or residents is an important aspect in the caring role and can promote a trusting relationship in future encounters.

While some service providers are embracing these changes and instituting new policies and practices, there is still a long way to go. Therefore, it is imperative that a supportive and positive environment be maintained to guarantee that sexual expression is identified as a basic tenet of life for the ageing person or couple within both the residential and the community environments.

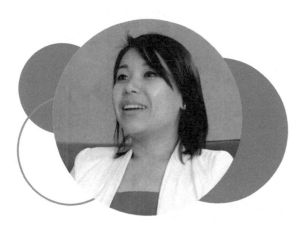

Dr Cindy's story

 Begin viewing Dr Cindy's story to 'Challenges and barriers to sexual expression' or read the transcript.

Dr Cindy begins by discussing the sexual construct and the differing view of sexuality. She goes on to give an example where younger people may have a specific view of when older people should and should not be having intimate relationships, and how they feel this should be expressed.

Reflection

Take the time to reflect on your own perceptions.

1. How old is too old to be having a sexual relationship?

2. Is there a time limit on when individuals should stop participating in a physical relationship?

3. Is sexuality merely a physical relationship? If not, what else does it encompass and how might this be expressed between individuals?

Myth or fact

Myths play a key role in shaping the way that we view the world. They may also impact on decision-making processes in work environments, staffing processes and care directives. It is important to be mindful of the difference between myth and reality. Here are some thought-provoking statements that may generate discussion between you and your colleagues. See if you can decide the myth from reality.

- It is not acceptable for older persons over the age of 75 to kiss in public places where they might be seen by others.
- Individuals over the age of 80 very rarely engage in the physical act of sexual intercourse and never perform oral sex with a partner.
- Elderly men over the age of 75 think less about sex than do women of the same age.
- There have been many studies about sexuality and the ageing population and these studies have proven that as the years increase, the willingness to think and engage in sexual expression is heightened due to the need for companionship and support.
- Individuals in their younger years (25 to 35) will experience more satisfaction in relation to their sexuality than those in the older population (i.e. over 55).
- The lesbian, gay, bisexual, transgender and intersex (LGBTI) community is just a group of people that dress up and belong to a cult.

Reflection

1. Can you tell the myth from reality? Did this generate discussion between you and your colleagues?

2. Can you think of any more myths that you may have heard about sexuality and the aged within your circle of friends and family?

3. How do you think these myths have evolved? What impact do you believe these myths might have on client care and service provision if they were taken up by a healthcare organisation?

4. What might be done to prevent or alter these perceptions within the local community or a healthcare setting?

Challenges and barriers to sexual expression

The desire to connect to another human both physically and emotionally is a natural state of being. Most individuals seek to be loved or to participate in a sexual or intimate relationship with another person. How this is expressed may vary from person to person and from relationship to relationship. Barriers to this may impede the wellbeing of the individual and affect their future physical and psychological health.

 Continue viewing Dr Cindy's story to 'Cognitive capacity to consent' or read the transcript.

Inquiry

Dr Cindy discusses these barriers as significant in preventing the person's expression of their own sexuality. She also supports the *Sexualities and Dementia: Education Resource for Health Professionals* provided by Queensland Dementia Training Study Centre (see the Further readings and references for this chapter at the end of the book for further details). Outline the barriers to sexual expression identified by Dr Cindy.

Action

A Choose two or three barriers to sexual expression and describe the impact they might have on someone in your care within the residential or community setting.

B Explore the concept of barriers to sexuality. How might these barriers facilitate negative outcomes for the client or resident and their family within the clinical setting, as well as impact on staffing workloads?

C Critically analyse the barriers to sexuality in relation to current changes in healthcare reform. What changes have been identified in recent months to ensure a better understanding of the individual's need for sexual expression in all its forms? How is this to be articulated within the care setting? What examples have you seen of this occurring within the workplace setting at present?

Inquiry

Bouman, Arcelus and Benbow (2006 and 2007) discuss the concept of sexuality in their Nottingham Study as they review both the literature and staff attitudes in relation to sexuality and ageing. Take the time to read these two articles as an example of contemporary literature available in this field of study.

Bouman WP, Arcelus J, Benbow SM 2006 Nottingham study of sexuality & ageing (NoSSA I). Attitudes regarding sexuality and older people: a review of the literature. Sexual and Relationship Therapy 21(2):149–161

www.tandfonline.com/doi/abs/10.1080/14681990600618879#.UszT80l-_mQ

Bouman WP, Arcelus J, Benbow SM 2007 Nottingham study of sexuality and ageing (NoSSA II). Attitudes of care staff regarding sexuality and residents: A study in residential and nursing homes. Sexual and Relationship Therapy 22(1):45–61

www.tandfonline.com/doi/abs/10.1080/146819900600637630#.UszTsUl-_mQ

Reflection

Reflect on what you have learned from the chapter so far. Also consider the perceptions of sexuality that you grew up with and those of your colleagues as you have worked your way through the chapter. After reading the articles in the Inquiry, answer the following questions.

1. Have your views changed in any way?
2. Are your views similar to or disparate from those given by the participants in the study?
3. Why might that be?

Sexuality and dementia

For those clients or residents who may be experiencing episodes of dementia, expressing their sexuality through intimacy (e.g. hugging, kissing and physical expressions of sexuality) may play an increasing role in their efforts to be more physically close to others as they lose touch with what has been familiar or known to them for so many years. Not only are they experiencing changes in their moods and memory but they are also not recognising familiar spousal or partner relationships that may have been longstanding.

This can be heartbreaking for family members and requires a sensitive approach to caring for both the client or resident and their partner. Behavioural changes during this time may become inappropriate and it is the healthcare professional's role to assess the difference between what is appropriate behaviour for the person and what may be inappropriate.

Dr Cindy discusses a case study in relation to an older resident with dementia and the staff's role in this experience.

 Continue viewing Dr Cindy's story to 'Current research into the need for intimacy and sexual expression' or read the transcript.

Reflection

1. Are there any events similar to this that you may have experienced within your clinical practice or your working life?

2. List any examples of inappropriate behaviour displayed by the resident or client as a trigger for your understanding of their need for sexual expression. You might also like to refer again to *Sexualities and Dementia: Education Resource for Health Professionals.*

3. Did other staff members, residents or clients, and family respond to this behaviour within the care setting positively or negatively?

4. Who, if anyone, did you call on for assistance? Or did you resolve this situation yourself?

5. Were family notified or involved in the situation and, if so, was this resolved to everyone's satisfaction?

6. If this was resolved, how was it resolved? If it was not, why?

Inquiry

Responding to the changing behaviours and needs of the resident or client who is experiencing dementia depends on knowledge of the individual's rights and responsibilities, their capacity to make informed decisions and your understanding of practical strategies to facilitate a positive outcome for all those involved. The resident's or client's behaviour may be triggered through diminishing capacity, so healthcare professionals need to be aware of the signs and symptoms of these changing stages and how these may manifest in sexual expression.

Ensuring a mutually satisfactory outcome for all involved is a complex care strategy and may require a number of care interventions based on an

understanding of legislative standards. These include rights and responsibilities, capacity, privacy, responsive measures, incident and risk management, reporting mechanisms, effective documentation and so on. Access the following documents to develop a better understanding.

Third party representatives—adults with a temporary or permanent incapacity, Australian Law Reform Commission

www.alrc.gov.au/publications/70.%20Third%20 Party%20Representatives/adults-temporary- or-permanent-incapacity

Aged Care Act 1997 (Cwlth)

www.comlaw.gov.au/Details/C2014C00316

Information Privacy Act 2009 (Qld)

www.qld.gov.au/law/your-rights/privacy-and-right- to-information/privacy-rights/

Action

Within the care setting, you might also experience unwanted advances from clients or residents. These experiences can be frightening, leaving staff feeling isolated and fearful of returning to work.

A Have you ever experienced a time when you felt that a resident or client approached you with unwanted advances? What did you do in this situation to ensure your own physical and emotional safety and that of the resident or client?

B Identify the triggers for unwanted sexual behaviours within a dementia-specific unit or facility. What strategies might you employ (i.e. care based, work practices, human resource) that will de-escalate the situation and prevent future episodes?

C Reflect on your current workplace (or one where you have recently been employed). What policies and procedures did the organisation or facility enact to respond to changes in the *Aged Care Act 1997*? How was this articulated to staff? How is this monitored during day-to-day practice?

The role of the healthcare professional

Your role is integral to ensuring best practice outcomes for residents and clients by ensuring that they may have a long and fulfilling life, as part of a relationship with another person. The healthcare professional should respond to the individual's need for sexuality through support for the person, whether that be in the community or within a residential care setting.

Further websites, videos and readings relevant to this subject have been provided for you in the Further readings and references at the end of the book.

 Finish viewing Dr Cindy's story or read the transcript.

Reflection

Take the time to reflect on your current role, either as a student or as a clinician within the workplace, and answer the following questions.

1. How is the concept of sexuality and sexual expression managed at the aged care facility, community organisation or hospital setting in which you are currently working?

2. Is sexuality managed differently for those clients living in the community setting than those residents located in a residential aged care facility? If so, why so?

3. How will staff respond to a family member when an older person finds a new partner and wishes to engage in a sexual relationship with them? Have you experienced this at your workplace? Was there a positive outcome to this interaction?

4. In her story, Dr Cindy discusses the difficulty older people have in discussing their needs in relation to sexuality. They are often fearful of the health professional's 'ageist' view and do not often know how to start the conversation. Staff often experience difficulty discussing issues and may falter when clients raise a number of personal issues. Outline the strategies you will use to ensure that clients or residents are put at ease and feel comfortable enough to discuss their sexuality without concern.

5. What training do health professionals need to give them the skills to provide appropriate support for these residents or clients?

6. How should healthcare professionals phrase questions to express an empathetic approach to care-driven solutions for the client or resident who might require support with sexual concerns?

7. Is different training required for staff caring for clients or residents within the LGBTI community? If so, what type of training?

8. How might the healthcare needs of clients or residents within the LGBTI community differ from others?

9. The LGBTI community has been identified as the 'hidden' community. Why is this? How will you respond to this concept in your day-to-day practice? How will you access this group to provide support or education (or promote services)?

10. What type of promotional or educational information is best suited to assist clients or residents to understand this topic? Is this readily available? If so, where would you access this information? If not, why not?

Inquiry

Staff from a multicultural background may find it difficult to deal with issues of sexuality if they come from a conservative, religious upbringing. The increase in the ageing population and the expectations of the baby boomer generation may make residential and community aged care look decidedly different in the future. Residents that are part of the LGBTI community may be sitting in the dining or lounge room waiting for their medication and staff will need to adjust to this. They may even request time with their partners.

Organisations need to become proactive rather than reactive to the changing face of healthcare. Policies and protocols must reflect the needs of the resident or client with clear guidelines that support the individual's choice to express themselves through intimacy and sexual relationships, whatever form that might take.

The Department of Social Services has reviewed its standards in light of the *Living Long, Living Better Health Reform 2012* to support an individual's choice in all aspects of their life, including sexual expression. Therefore, it is the duty of healthcare service providers to ensure that they respond to this effectively through policy development, process implementation, education, training and service facilitation that reflects client choices.

Action

A Have your views on sexuality and ageing changed now that you have completed this chapter? What role can you play in your future career as an aged care worker to support clients and residents to express their sexuality?

B Review the current organisational aged policies and practices within a defined care environment in which you have either worked or attended on clinical placement. How do they address sexual expression within healthcare services? Are there defined and observable examples of theory in practice within the workplace?

C Explore the current literature and healthcare legislation in relation to sexuality and ageing.

Critically analyse how this contemporary information has impacted on the local organisational decision-making policies and procedures in relation to the choice of sexual expression by clients and residents. Has the LGBTI legislation been incorporated within these policies and processes? If not, outline a plan to do so.

A FINAL WORD

Dr Cindy is a specialist in the field of sexuality and ageing, and an expert in research into sexuality and dementia. She is passionate about staff education and training in this area, and is willing to share her knowledge and skill with others to ensure best practice outcomes for clients and residents.

While policies and procedures guide care, the role of staff and carers is paramount to providing optimal service and lifestyle choices. Both the story and the associated literature reinforces this notion and emphasises the importance of a deeper understanding of these concepts. It is imperative that healthcare professionals remain aware of the ever-changing needs of the ageing population, as notions of sexuality evolve in line with community expectations and values. Only through ongoing education and training may we all keep up to date with contemporary practice that benefits clients and residents.

CHAPTER 6

The Sandwich Generation

INTRODUCTION

This chapter introduces you to the 'sandwich generation'. This is the generation of people who care for the generation above them and the generations below. This term was coined in the 1980s by Dorothy Miller, a researcher who used the term to refer to inequality in the exchange of resources and support between generations (Raphael & Schlesinger, 1994). Specifically, Miller was referring to a segment of the middle-aged generation that provides support to both young and older family members yet does not receive reciprocal support in exchange. However, we are using this term to merely identify the group of people who provide intergenerational care.

This chapter refers to two videos of women who speak about their roles within this sandwich generation. Each woman tells their stories about what their roles in life have been and are now. Theresa is a nurse who works full-time. She cares for her mother, her son and her grandchild. Barbara is 71 years old. She cared for her son who has quadriplegia, her nieces and nephews, as well as her aunt. These women take you through their journeys with an honesty that is enlightening.

Listening to these stories will also give you the opportunity to reflect on your own knowledge and opinions in relation to the difficulties, challenges and highlights of being a carer for multiple generations.

Before you begin ... How perceptions shape ideas of families undertaking care

Before you begin, think about your own views of the people who undertake caring activities within the community. Think critically about how you perceive them. Have you ever considered them within the sandwich generation framework? The following are some of the issues you will need to consider.

- Do they do these caring activities because family are involved? Should they have to do this?

- What would happen to the healthcare system or other community support resources if they decided to hand over these roles to recognised community agencies of care?

- Should they be formally recognised and offered training for their carer activities?

- Should there be more government involvement; for example, supervision, financial reimbursement and accountability?

- How many people are undertaking these roles? Do we just see the 'tip of the iceberg'?

- Many of these sandwich carers are older themselves. Is it fair that they should be undertaking all this ongoing and often stressful work?

The aim of this chapter is not to provide you with definitive answers but to introduce you to the notion of sandwich generation carers and to encourage you to do more research in this area, especially where your professional practice involves sandwich generation carers.

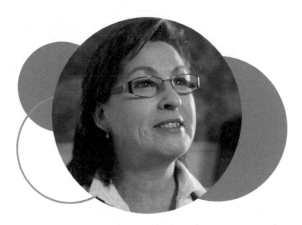

Theresa's story

 View Theresa's story or read the transcript.

Reflection

As you think about Theresa's story, try and consider what it must mean for her to be caring for her mother and son, working full-time as well as trying to look after herself.

1. What do you believe are her main challenges?
2. What would happen to the following if Theresa was not able to do this caring:
   a. her son?
   b. Theresa's personal values and concepts of family?
3. What would happen to Theresa's mother if Theresa was unable to provide support and care?

Who is the sandwich generation?

As identified by Miller, the sandwich generation is the generation of people who care for the generation above them and the generations below. That is, they are generally caring for their older parents or relatives while supporting their own children. They are therefore sitting in the middle of two (and

sometimes more) needy groups of people. Although not always, they are often women.

The sandwich generation provides considerable amount of holistic care to both generations. This includes practical care such as bathing and grooming, maintenance of life activities such as assistance with shopping, doctors' visits and housework plus a considerable amount of emotional support. As Theresa advises us in her story, the carer is often torn between responsibilities and is frequently emotionally tired.

Anecdotally, they are often seen as being between the ages of 40 and 60; however, in practice they are often much older. They are frequently seen by others as being older people themselves and as they also age, there is less time and opportunity for them to consider their own needs.

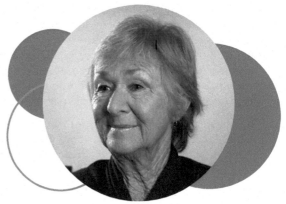

Barbara's story

 View Barbara's story or read the transcript.

Reflection

As you would have heard, Barbara has multiple responsibilities. She undertook all personal care activities for her adult son who lived with her, she cares for an older aunt and she also cares for nieces and nephews.

1. Is it right/wrong to expect Barbara to provide cross-generational care for her family?
2. Should Barbara be offered more assistance?
3. Barbara is now 71 years old. Is there an age when undertaking so much care is too much?

Inquiry

While listening to the stories, you will have noted that Barbara and Theresa undertake a considerable amount of work caring for both the younger generation and the older generation between which they are sandwiched. In each story, some extra care was offered and taken. However, this added care was not always successful. While we have a system of home and community care that is mandated to help support individuals within the home and community environment, questions can still be asked.

1. Does the sandwich generation require some sort of help or assistance?
2. Who should offer this help?
3. What help should be offered if it was needed?
4. Is the help we offer appropriate?

Action

A Choose three commonalities of a person who is deemed to be part of the sandwich generation. Using these commonalities, briefly explain who the sandwich generation is and what their challenges may be.

B Explore issues related to the sandwich generation and consider how the care given by the sandwich generation affects the health and/or community care systems within our society. Is it positive or negative? Justify your responses.

C Considering the changing population demographics of our society, critically analyse the role of the sandwich generation carer and consider future burdens or impacts that may occur based on population trends. How can we prepare for these changes? You will need to undertake some self-directed research into population trends to complete this.

Readings

Pause at this moment and read the following articles. They will give you an overview of the sandwich generation. Although The Family Squeeze is only the first chapter of a book, it provides an easy-to-read outline of the sandwich generation carer. Note the obvious similarities between Barbara's and Theresa's stories. The *Sydney Morning Herald* article contains case studies of people with similar stories. Also view the YouTube clip.

The sandwich generation

www.hands-in-service.com/sandwich-generation.html

The sandwich generation impact

http://hisinarizona.wix.com/sgimpact#!logistics/c7ms

Kingsmill S, Schlesinger B 1998 The family squeeze: surviving the sandwich generation. University of Toronto, Canada

http://books.google.com.au/books?hl=en&lr=&id=eOx0hkn4i1AC&oi=fnd&pg=PR9&dq=the+sandwich+generation&ots=O8lotMu1p0&sig=gWmDZXJwepUgj0yUC6hJ9H65ksc#v=onepage&q=the%20sandwich%20generation&f=false

Power, J 28 July 2012 The sandwich generation. Sydney Morning Herald

www.smh.com.au/national/the-sandwich-generation-20120727-22zj2.html

Are you caught in the sandwich generation?

www.youtube.com/watch?v=bCBoeBrZ4KU

What is the burden for the sandwich generation?

Sandwich generation carers provide a holistic service to their families, covering a whole spectrum of needs. While they may be providing personal care to one generation, they will also have to provide care to the other generation. Consider Barbara's story; she was her quadriplegic son's personal carer as well as providing care for an older aunt and often other family members. Theresa too spoke of the care she had to give her mother as well as the care she needed to give her son. Both these women had multiple roles that were often fluid and extended to more than just one member of each generation. This is anecdotally identified as a pattern that will often occur with other sandwich generation carers.

Let's briefly consider the burden on a person who is a sandwich generation carer. Obviously there is going to be a change in family dynamics. For example, where once the mother cared for the daughter, the situation has reversed and the daughter is now caring for the mother. This change in dynamics could have serious implications for the whole family.

As the person ages, they will not have the same physical capabilities to undertake personal care activities. Barbara was still showering and toileting her severely disabled son in her late sixties. Theresa was undertaking personal care activities for her mother in her fifties. They had minimal respite from these activities, even in the face of any personal physical challenges. As both Theresa and Barbara are deemed to be older women, we have situations in which older people are undertaking activities that many women younger would not wish to do from a physical perspective.

There is also no emotional respite for these carers. Theresa speaks of how at times it becomes quite emotional and stressful and sometimes feels as though she '… can't do this anymore'. Barbara spoke about feeling that she '… had to keep going. I didn't have any choices'.

While neither Barbara nor Theresa spoke of the *financial* burden of caring, it too is an important component of sandwich generation care. As caring will often impact on the ability of the sandwich generation carer to undertake full-time paid roles, their ability to have an appropriate financial reserve will be difficult to achieve. Not being able to build sufficient superannuation funds to help support their retirement will become problematic in later years.

Readings

The following articles will help you understand the importance of carers and start considering the burden on them. In the Submission to the Productivity Commission Inquiry into Caring for Older Australians, read carefully through the sections that identify the importance of the family in caring. The YouTube clip is a light-hearted look at the sandwich generation, but very clearly identifies some of the stressors which contribute to the burden of care.

Carers Australia May 2008 Submission to the National Health and Hospitals Reform Commission

www.health.gov.au/internet/nhhrc/publishing.nsf/Content/055-ca/$FILE/Submissions%20055%20-%20Carers%20Australia%20Submission.pdf (Read paragraph 7.)

Carers Australia July 2010 Submission to the Productivity Commission Inquiry into Caring for Older Australians

www.carersaustralia.com.au/storage/Submission-to-PC-Caring-Older-Australians.pdf

Broderick E 2013 Caring for the carers. The Australian

www.theaustralian.com.au/national-affairs/opinion/caring-for-the-carers/story-e6frgd0x-1226585430408#

Living with integrity: the sandwich generation http://www.youtube.com/watch?v=OoLgfRNW124

Inquiry

Considering the burden on sandwich generation carers, there is an extremely strong potential for the

carer to need help and assistance at some point. This is not unforeseeable. However, in the videos of Theresa and Barbara, neither felt that what they were doing was too much to manage. They did not see what they do as a burden. This does not mean that we should not provide support and care for the sandwich generation of carers.

There are a number of supporting websites that offer basic advice to carers about caring for themselves, but are these enough?

Read the following articles and view the YouTube clip that have been developed for carers. Reflect upon whether they fulfil the needs of sandwich generation carers.

Caring for yourself while caring for others: fact sheet

https://au.reachout.com/Factsheets/C/Caring-for-yourself-while-caring-for-others#other

Carer Allowance

www.humanservices.gov.au/customer/services/centrelink/carer-allowance

Tips for carers to take care of themselves (p 4)

www.humanservices.gov.au/spw/customer/publications/resources/cd011/cd011-1305en.pdf

Improving family dynamics with in-home care

www.caringnews.com/pub.59/issue.1741/

Caregiving Club me time Monday sandwich generation tips

www.youtube.com/watch?v=Hpg405JhJHg

Action

There needs to be a policy of best practice in supporting the sandwich generation. This policy must be supported by a plan of action that is reasonable and achievable. Undertake the following activities in relation to the experiences of either Theresa or Barbara.

A Consider the changing needs of Barbara or Theresa as they age and maintain their sandwich generation carer role. How could an in-home carer provide them with support? Consider both physical and emotional needs.

B Consider the change of family dynamics that occurs when one generation takes over the care of others. How do you perceive this will affect family relationships? How can this be assisted by the health professional? Should professional psychologists, counsellors and other relevant team members become involved at any early stage? Or should they wait and provide crisis intervention when required?

C Identify how, at an organisational level (government and non-government), policies and practices could be developed and implemented to support sandwich generation carers within the community. How would you identify who were undertaking these care practices? How would you ensure that they become aware of any programs that could help ease their burdens of care?

Reflection

1. Is there a burden of care for sandwich generation carers, or do they undertake their caring responsibilities as part of their role and responsibilities?
2. Should there be government and agency policies to advise and assist these carers in a more robust manner?
3. What can be done practically to minimise this burden?

A FINAL WORD

This chapter has discussed the burden of care for the sandwich generation carer. With multiple responsibilities and often limited time for themselves, they face a number of challenges of their own.

Changing family dynamics, physical challenges linked to their own ageing, and emotional stressors are just a few of these challenges. While we have seen that there is acknowledgement for their role and recognition for the amount of care that they administer, there seems to be minimal help and support for them. Although they will often just 'get on with the business of caring', they will frequently do so from a sense of duty and in the knowledge that 'it has to be done'. Could the burden of care be lessened for these carers if they were given better choices?

By now you should have a thorough understanding of the concept of the sandwich generation and what it means to the individual. However, it does not stop there with a new term being coined: 'the club sandwich generation'. This refers to the phenomena of caring for three or more generations, due to continuously changing demographics. Consider Barbara's story—perhaps she typifies a club sandwich generation carer as she cares for one generation older and two generations younger than her.

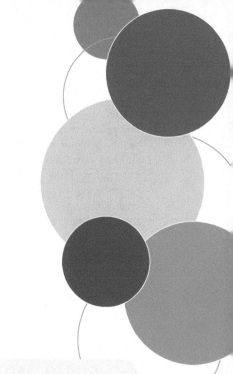

CHAPTER 7

Maintaining Independence in the Home

INTRODUCTION

This chapter takes you on the journey from the manager's story of working with staff and supporting people who wish to remain living within their home, to the clinician's story as she manages the day-to-day care of the client in the community, then to a woman who tells her story as she maintains a sense of independence within her community.

The first story is told by Wendy, a community service manager with 30 years experience as a registered nurse. She has managed a range of services for frail aged clients living in the community, those living with carers, some living alone and many living with dementia.

Roseanne, a registered nurse, then tells her story of working for over 23 years within the community setting providing daily care for frail aged clients and their families who wish to remain independent in their own homes.

The third story in recounted by Barbara. Barbara is a 91-year-old woman who lives alone in her own home. Despite the challenges associated with being older and alone, she strives hard to retain her independence within her own home.

Before you begin … How perceptions of maintaining independence as we age shape practice

Think about those older people currently living in the community. Many individuals live at home quite independently or with minimal support from family, friends or community groups. Continued community and social connectedness is a positive outcome for the ageing person, enhancing their physical, psychological, social, emotional and spiritual wellbeing. For some individuals, however, the burden of care becomes too great to be able to maintain an independent lifestyle without assistance. For most, this assistance may come from a range of support

services that result in long-term, achievable outcomes and are available from healthcare providers. It is important to understand available services, not just consider them in the event of a crisis.

- Would you know what to look for if you needed assistance at home?

- Would you know where to access services for a family member if you needed them urgently?

- Who would you ask to assist you with your enquiries?

- What information or paperwork is required to enable you to access services?

- What do these services cost?

- If you have a family member who is deteriorating at home should you consider community services or is it better to place them in a residential facility? On what information/ considerations should your decision be based?

Maintaining independence within one's home is highly desirable for most individuals. The Australian Institute of Health and Welfare (AIHW) provides a range of information on the internet within their Aged care data cubes which outline the latest statistics and publications on older persons either living within the community or choosing to enter residential care. Take the time to go to this website and do your own search.

Australian Institute of Health and Welfare, Australian Government

www.aihw.gov.au/aged-care-data-cubes/#rac2010

It is important to remember that all services available to individuals and their carers need to be person-centred and based on personal choice. Now watch as Wendy tells the story of managing services within the community setting.

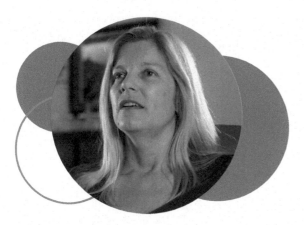

Wendy's story

 Begin viewing Wendy's story to 'Access to services' or read the transcript.

Reflection

Wendy discusses the range and types of services available and the complexity of the healthcare professional's involvement in managing equipment, providing care, partnership arrangements, financial accountability and family enablement in this process. Reflect on the following questions, either on your own or with a colleague, and identify the key issues

in the video that you wish to focus on for further learning.

1. Outline the different services Wendy identified as being available to individuals living within the community and that might enable them to live independently in their own home.

2. How might these services facilitate a better lifestyle outcome for the person and their family?

3. What equipment might be necessary to support a client and family when a person is living in their own home? How might this be accessed (e.g. purchased, borrowed or hired)?

4. What would be the benefits of working with other organisations to care for individuals living in the community?

5. Highlight the financial issues that might affect the client, carer and family when accessing community services.

Accessing services

Accessing appropriate services when needed is the key to ensuring individuals living in the community can maintain a quality lifestyle for as long as possible. It is imperative that healthcare professionals understand how to do this. You should know what is available for each person, how to refer that person to the services that will best suit their needs and how these services will transition as the person's needs change over time.

Access points are available to meet an individual's needs, depending on criteria linked to eligibility and support needs. The Further readings and references for this chapter will help you to better understand the range of information available for people and healthcare professionals wishing to source services for individuals wanting to remain at home.

Queensland Aged Care Assessment Team contacts

https://www.agedcareguide.com.au/acats. asp?stateid=4

Queensland Government, Access to community care services

www.qld.gov.au/community/getting-support-health-social-issue/access-community-care-services

 Continue viewing Wendy's story to 'Challenges working in the community' or read the transcript.

Listen to Wendy's discussion about the following issues in relation to accessing services:

- waiting lists
- service provision types
- assessment criteria
- partnering with other organisations
- packages available
- costs involved in care.

Reflection

1. How important is it to undertake early assessment and planning in the care of the individual?

2. If you are managing the service, what specific information would you need to be aware of in relation to the service type?

3. What specific information will you need to be aware of in relation to the care needs of the client and the family?

4. What issues might arise with staff working autonomously within the community?

5. How might volunteers assist with the overall functioning of the service?

6. What is the impact of cost when clients are considering whether to take up services?

7. How would you know if there were any gaps in current services? What information, tools or resources would you use to identify these gaps? How would you manage these gaps in services that you identify to ensure that you get the best possible outcome for your clients and family or carers?

Inquiry

It is essential that community managers and healthcare professionals are familiar with current legislation and the guidelines that reflect these initiatives. The manager's role is to participate in policy development and constantly review processes within the local organisation as changes occur. Remaining aware of government changes may have a positive or negative impact on the workplace, as Wendy outlines two examples: workplace health and safety, and policy standards and staff difficulties in saying 'no'.

 Finish viewing Wendy's story or read the transcript.

Evolving societal and demographic shifts in healthcare, as well as the increased ageing population, has led to Commonwealth aged care reform. The development and implementation of the Living Longer Living Better key initiatives provide the footprint for future aged care services. Review the information relevant to community services, which clarifies the future direction of consumer-directed care and the government's proposal for healthy living for an ageing population.

Department of Social Services, Aged care reform

www.dss.gov.au/our-responsibilities/ageing-and-aged-care/aged-care-reform

Another source of information is the Home Care Standards. These standards are a foundation on which all community services are measured and ensure organisations provide equitable, measurable outcomes for all clients who receive community services.

Department of Health, Home care standards and quality reporting documentation

https://www.health.gov.au/internet/main/publishing.nsf/Content/ageing-commcare-qualrep-standards.htm

Action

A Describe the types of services available to individuals so that they are able to remain living independently within their home. How are these services helpful to the person, their carer and their family?

B Explore the complexity of access and equity in relation to service provision across the community services in your area. How might this be affected by funding, staffing ratios and organisational policies and processes? What would be your role as a manager in addressing these factors? Outline the steps that you might take.

C Review the current changes in Australian government legislation in relation to consumer-directed care, client choice and the seamless approach to healthcare services. Consider the policies within your organisation in line with this legislation. Critically analyse the gaps between current policy and new legislation, and map out a plan for improvement.

The clinician

The role of the healthcare professional in assisting the individual and family to remain safe and independent at home is an important one. This person provides not only practical day-to-day service provision but also information, education, counselling, advocacy and support to the client, carer and family.

As the second story unfolds, Roseanne discusses her 23 years of experience as a registered nurse working with the frail aged within the community setting. Her passion as a clinician is evident as she outlines the importance of understanding the intricate role of the nurse within this setting.

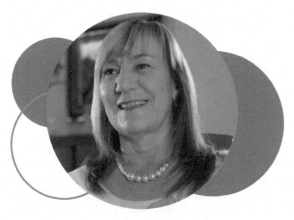

Roseanne's story

 Begin viewing Roseanne's story to 'How clients access the services' or read the transcript.

Reflection

Consider the variety of services available in the community, the number of service types and the range of funding. Roseanne has highlighted the different services and the types of funding for each service. Reflect on your knowledge of what is available to people living in your community and what would be available to you or a family member if you needed to access services.

- What services are available in your local area that you and your family might access?
- What does the term 'service type' mean and what are some of the examples that Roseanne used in the video?
- What are the different funded services that people may access when seeking support to remain independently in their own home as they age?

- Are there different service types linked to different funding streams, and if so how are these identified?
- Where would you access this information?

Community access and consent

Individuals, carers and family members access services via a range of portals, both formal and informal. As mentioned previously, the access point is a gateway to service access. However, there are a variety of ways to enter a service. Needs identification plays a pivotal role in providing the appropriate service for safe and independent quality of life for the aged person who wishes to remain living at home.

As part of her story, Roseanne outlines a number of methods for accessing services and identifies the range and types of activities that she performs on a day-to-day basis in her clinical role. She highlights the impact of isolation on elderly individuals who risk living alone without appropriate community service access and stresses the need for appropriate care planning and service integration.

Consent to care is a significant factor in establishing successful, streamlined quality service provision. The concept of consent should be fully explained to the client by the healthcare professional as part of the admissions process when a person wishes to receive community services. Everyone needs to be aware that the right to take up or refuse services is a choice that the individual is able to make at any time throughout the life of the service.

 Continue viewing Roseanne's story to 'Delegation of care and decision-making' or read the transcript.

You may wish to research the concept of consent further by searching the internet or reading the chapter on consent in the text below.

Staunton P, Chiarella M 2012 Law for Nurses and Midwives, 7th edn. Churchill Livingstone, Australia

Reflection

As you listen to Roseanne's story, consider the essential aspects of the registered nurse's role in this setting. A number of times Roseanne mentions the importance of a comprehensive assessment, as well as specific tasks that she undertakes as part of her working day. Reflect on the following questions and either consider the answers individually or discuss them with a colleague.

1. How important is it to undertake a comprehensive assessment for a client being admitted into the community service?

2. What will this information tell you?

3. How important is it to ensure that the comprehensive assessment links to effective care planning? How will you ensure that this occurs?

4. Roseanne has identified a range of tasks she may undertake each day. Can you think of any others that she has not mentioned? What are they?

5. How might you measure the success of the care that you are providing for a client and/or family within the community setting?

6. What are the environmental issues that you will need to consider when caring for an individual and their family in a community setting?

Inquiry

Effective documentation is an important component of the healthcare professional's role. Roseanne shares the significance of documentation and outlines this as a method for communicating the day-to-day record of client care to all members of the community team. Healthcare documentation provides a reference point from which all past, current and future care may be translated and it enables members of the team to develop an understanding of what is required to achieve best practice outcomes for the client and his or her family.

Australia currently has the following health record management guidelines that organisations can access and implement as part of policy and process within the workplace. These may be accessed at www.standards.org.au.

- AS/NZS ISO 30300-2012 Management systems for recordkeeping—fundamentals and vocabulary
- AS/NZS ISO 30301-2012 Management systems for recordkeeping—requirements

Also consider reading the following article which outlines a study undertaken within the Australian aged care setting and reflects on the relationship between the registered nurse's knowledge of nursing documentation, the documentation process and the outcomes of documentation within aged care. Results identified not only the importance of appropriate documentation but the need for a

comprehensive education program that enhances the health professional's skill in documentation.

Daskein R, Moyle W, Creedy D 2009 Aged-care nurses' knowledge of nursing documentation: an Australian perspective. Journal of Clinical Nursing 18(14):2087–2095

Continue with Roseanne's story as she discusses the issue of delegation of care and her responsibilities as a registered nurse when working with a range of healthcare staff.

Delegation of duties

 Continue viewing Roseanne's story to 'Meeting client expectations: case study' or read the transcript.

Reflection

Consider what you know about your scope of practice and your current role as a student or as a staff member within the workplace.

1. If you are currently registered with a national body such as the Australian Health Practitioner Regulation Agency (AHPRA), what does this imply? What are or what will be your requirements to practice?

2. What does it mean to function within your 'scope of practice'?

3. Do you know how to access the codes and guidelines that reflect your particular healthcare profession?

4. What are your responsibilities in relation to the delegation of duties under your decision-making framework according to your registration requirements?

5. Where would you go to access this information?

6. If you are a community care worker and supervised by a registered nurse, what is your responsibility in relation to notification of client issues? When might you discuss issues of concern with the registered nurse?

Inquiry

You might like to take the time to access the resources available to you and read further in relation to scope of practice and delegation.

Australian Health Practitioner Regulation Agency (AHPRA)

www.ahpra.gov.au

Fact sheet: scope of practice for registered nurses and midwives

www.nursingmidwiferyboard.gov.au/Codes-Guidelines-Statements/FAQ/Scope-of-practice-for-registered-nurses-and-midwives.aspx

Nursing and Midwifery Board of Australia Codes and Guidelines

www.nursingmidwiferyboard.gov.au/Codes-Guidelines-Statements/Codes-Guidelines.aspx%23nurses

Community in the future

Contemporary health planning has meant a shift from organisation-driven service provision to that of client-focused care to involve clients in all decisions, including service types, choice of service providers, timeframes for service delivery and willingness to pay for that service. This new model of care has brought about a sense of tentativeness from organisations as management wades through the minefield of rosters, costs and service remodelling.

For consumers, it will mean a re-education in accessing services, understanding the range of services available, self-managing budgets, and choice and decision making in relation to service providers. Healthcare providers will need to develop enhanced skills in communication and negotiation, while ensuring that the expectations of both the organisation and the consumer are met to everyone's satisfaction.

Roseanne next outlines a case study related to a frail aged client where family involvement, negotiation in relation to care and expectations play a key role in the final outcome for the client.

 Finish viewing Roseanne's story or read the transcript.

Action

Now consider your own role as a novice or practising registered nurse within the healthcare setting.

A Describe the tasks that you may be asked to undertake to support clients, carers and their families within the community. What knowledge and skills will you need to have or develop to ensure that you are able to undertake these tasks in a safe and competent manner? Outline the

resources you may access to enable you to develop the knowledge and skills in this area.

B Explore the registered nurse's role within the community setting. How does this differ from that of a nurse within the acute care setting? What are the expectations or limitations of this role and the additional skills that may be required to support this role? Outline your understanding of a comprehensive assessment and how this links to developing a service plan that provides measurable outcomes within a consumer-directed model for clients and carers in the community setting.

C Review the current changes to the Home Care Package funding allocation. Consider the impacts of this on future allocation of services across community settings, in light of the ageing population and an individual's ability to maintain independence in their own home. Identify any service enhancements that will support this growing ageing population and changes to packaged care.

Living in the community

The next story is from Barbara, who aims to remain as independent as possible as an older person living in the community. As Barbara tells her story, you will hear how important it is for her to stay in her own home.

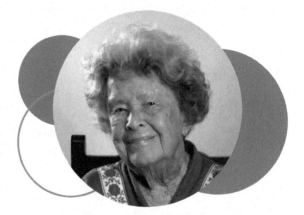

Barbara's story

 View Barbara's story or read the transcript.

Reflection

As you listen to Barbara's story, remember that she is 91 years old and has a degree of fragility which includes some mobility issues. There is no doubt that she can be seen as vulnerable. Ask yourself the following questions.

1. How safe is Barbara living alone in her own home?

2. Should she be allowed to stay at home alone?

3. Should there be more responsibility for healthcare professionals to strongly encourage women such as Barbara to move to a safer environment?

4. What additional healthcare services could be provided for Barbara to help her stay at home safely?

5. How have the community services enabled Barbara to remain within her own home?

Inquiry

Individuals have the right to choose how they wish to spend their older years and where they wish to live. They also have a right to live safely and be well supported within this environment. You have now viewed stories from both Wendy and Roseanne about the services that may be provided to community members. However, even though these services are available (at times) for the older person, they are not always well received or even wanted. Why is that? Also, many people living in the community are unsure how to access these services. Why?

Barbara has chosen to receive some services but does not wish to receive 'too much' in the way of intervention. Who should make the decision on how much service to give? Are there any contributing factors? Remember that without the interventions that are offered to Barbara it may be quite difficult for her to live safely within her own home. However, by remaining within her own home Barbara is far more content, happy, independent and in control.

Action

Consider Barbara's story and how the concepts she has discussed relate to maintaining independence at home.

A Is Barbara being given the necessary support to stay within her home? Briefly outline the other services that could be provided to Barbara.

B Barbara does not want to go into a nursing home; however, she is becoming increasingly frail. Is there ever a need to 'strongly' persuade a person to move into a nursing home? *Outside* of forced removal by regulation, outline any justifications that you may have for encouraging Barbara to take up a nursing home placement. How would you do this?

C Barbara is strongly independent and is receiving some family and health service support. Explain where family responsibility, community responsibility and government responsibility converge and diverge. How should those involved determine responsibilities of care?

A FINAL WORD

The role of the healthcare professional within the community is complex and diverse. Wendy and Roseanne are passionate about being healthcare professionals within the community setting, ensuring that their clients are able to maintain a fulfilling and independent lifestyle within their community. Roseanne reiterates this at the end of her story when she says that the best possible solution to her day is when she can ensure that they live a 'quality life' and has contributed to this.

In addition, Barbara comments that being able to maintain a lifestyle that enables her to stay in her own home for as long as possible is an essential component for her continuing health and wellbeing. As healthcare professionals, it is imperative that you have a working knowledge of the services, referral process, comprehensive assessment and care planning requirements to meet the growing needs of the ageing population to enable them to live successfully in their own home for as long as possible.

CHAPTER 8

Ageing and Health Compromise

INTRODUCTION

This chapter introduces you to some issues related to health compromise that can occur as the person ages. A health compromise is any condition that prevents or interferes with the body being able to function optimally. Health compromises become more frequent as we age due to a number of factors. These include the general deterioration of body structure and function, an increased inability for our bodies to respond to ill health and, at times, a lack of resources or opportunities to manage them.

Within this chapter are videos of three people who speak about quite different aspects of health compromise for the older person. Each of them also shares their experiences. Robert is a 66-year-old healthcare consumer who has suffered from chronic back pain since he was involved in an accident in his youth. He shares with us how his perceptions and pain management techniques change as he ages. Leonie is a naturopath and shares her stories about practising her profession with the older person. Her unique experiences provide insight into how the older person considers alternate health advice. Judy is a registered nurse who practises within the aged care environment. Her stories offer insight into issues associated with delirium, cognitive impairment and the older person.

Listening to these stories will also give you the opportunity to reflect on your own knowledge and opinions in relation to health compromises and ageing.

Before you begin ... How perceptions of health and health management can shape practice

Before you begin, think about your own views of the older person and health compromises. Is there a difference between sickness and ill health for the older person? Or are health compromises merely part of the degenerative processes associated with ageing? The following are some of the issues you will need to consider.

- Do you consider yourself old?
- How does a health compromise affect an older person?

- Are management strategies the same for an older person as they are for a younger one?
- How should health compromises be managed?
- Who owns the issues and management of health compromises? Is it the healthcare team or is it the person?
- Is offering consumer-directed care the appropriate way care for an older person with a health compromise?
- Is there a place for complementary therapies in managing health compromises?
- How do we ensure that the client receives the correct care?

The aim of this chapter is not to provide you with definitive answers but to introduce you to some of the issues that surround health compromises

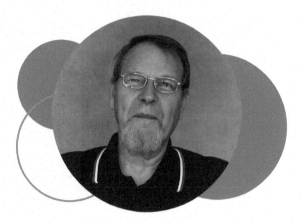

Robert's story

 View Robert's story or read the transcript.

Robert has been living with chronic pain for most of his life. Now as he ages and moves into his older years, he finds himself considering what he needs to do to manage his pain. He also shares his thoughts about the healthcare profession. Listen carefully to what he has to say about his experiences with healthcare professionals.

Reflection

1. What do you believe are the main issues that concern Robert?

   a. His lack of ability to move around freely?

   b. The constant chronic pain that he is in?

   c. His frustrations with healthcare professionals?

   d. Or is there something else that he considers to be his main concern?

As Robert has shared with us, a health compromise at a later age does not always have to be caused by the degeneration or decreased ability of our bodies to maintain a normal healthy environment. In his case, the compromise was caused by an incident that occurred when he was much younger. The damage that occurred then has slowly increased over the years.

As you would have heard in the My Story section of the video, he does question his decision-making choices following his accident and suggests that if he had followed a different path of treatment at that time, perhaps things may be different for him now. However, having lived with his pain for so long, he knows what works and what does not. Consider his

frustrations at having to explain repeatedly to health professionals what is wrong and what works, and being offered advice for treatment in which he has little faith.

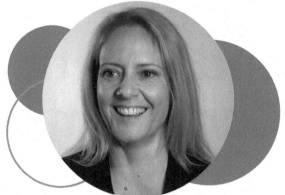

Leonie's story

 View Leonie's story or read the transcript.

Leonie is a practising naturopath and although she works with people of all ages, she undertakes considerable work with older people. She speaks earnestly about her belief that naturopaths should be working alongside mainstream health professionals. She also clearly articulates her view that many of a person's health compromises can be linked to diet and poor nutrition. Her story about the woman living in an aged care facility clearly identifies how she is able to improve health merely by including dietary supplements that resembled the diet of her youth.

Reflection

The provision of healthcare is frequently built on science that considers new technologies and/or treatments. Consider how that fits with a far more natural model of care that strips everything back to meeting basic needs.

1. Should the healthcare system be adapted to ensure that complementary therapies such as naturopathy are routinely included within our diagnosis and care planning cycles?

2. Should we consider the nutritional practices of older people when planning their care?

3. Is Leonie correct when she speaks about the importance of dietary supplements and simple

measures such as drinking more water, eating natural food and simply making sure that we have time to really listen to what our older people are saying to us? Or is this too simplistic an approach to care?

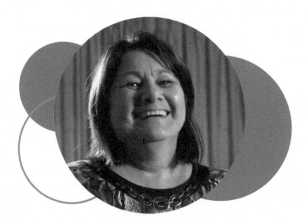

Judy's story

 View Judy's story or read the transcript.

Judy is a health professional and works with a considerable number of older people. She shares with us her stories about a significant health compromise that can have very serious consequences for the older person. Listen carefully as she discusses delirium and how it can be misdiagnosed for a number of other conditions. She stresses how important it is to get the diagnosis correct and to treat delirium appropriately. As she states, 'the sooner it [delirium] is found and treated, the better the outcomes are for the person'. Judy identifies the importance of getting support from the person's carer to help not only diagnose, but manage the care of the older person. She also discusses the importance of considering the basic and simple measures of assisting someone rather than always using pharmacological intervention as the forefront of management.

Reflection

1. How can we differentiate between dementia and delirium if we cannot gain a good history from the client?
2. What have you personally been taught in relation to caring for somebody who exhibits signs of delirium or confusion or agitation?

3. Do we always consider the most basic and simple measures within our care before we look at more complex strategies?

In the case study section, Judy tells the story of a patient who became agitated and how the attending healthcare team members wanted to treat her for this. Listen to the strength in her voice when she speaks about how she advised them to try simple measures first.

Inquiry

While listening to these stories, you will note that one common theme is that people want to take control of their own healthcare and decisions. Robert very clearly expressed his frustrations with the healthcare team in having to continuously repeat himself. He also spoke of his wish to 'continue and manage it [his pain] myself this way'. Leonie also spoke about the older people she works with and how they too often need someone to just listen to their concerns.

There are times when the healthcare team or the experts in healthcare are seen as 'holding the knowledge' and do not consider the knowledge people have about themselves. We ask people questions, develop a diagnosis and set a treatment plan. Continually asking Robert questions and developing plans that did not suit him contributed significantly to him turning away from the health profession in order to pursue his own course of treatments.

Within healthcare we move from various cycles of management. 'Consumer-centred care' was once the 'buzz' term for caring for our clients. However, you will find the term 'consumer-directed care' is now being used frequently. This is especially so for those living in the community and receiving help to maintain their independence.

There is a significant difference between these two models of care. Consumer-centred care has the client as the main focus: not a collection of body parts but a holistic person with emotions, beliefs and feelings that are unique to them. In consumer-centred care, we consult with the client to ensure that what we wish to do in terms of caring is what they want. We approach the client and, with their help, we design the interventions and support required.

However, consumer-directed care is aimed at ensuring that the client determines what types of care or services they need and who will deliver these. This ensures that the client receives the type of care and support that they choose and, importantly, it enables them to decide who is to deliver their care.

It is imperative to note that when using a consumer-directed model of care, it does not negate the need to ensure that the client is still the centre of our caring processes. The process of care becomes a two-tier model: the consumer directs their own care and chooses their own service providers, and then the chosen service providers plan and manage the care provided within a consumer-centred model in consultation with the client.

It is important also to consider the beliefs and practices with which many of our older people will have grown up. To them the doctor was often seen as the holder of the knowledge and that it would be most inappropriate for them to even suggest to a medical person what they believed they wanted or to make a decision about who they would like to care for them. Consumer-directed care and even consumer-centred care may cause them some anxiety in having to make these decisions.

Action

A If you were part of a team that was caring for Robert, how would you and/or your team assist him to manage his pain? What would be your approach? What strategies would you use? How would you ensure that he was an active participant in his care?

B Often the client is not fully advised of all the appropriate choices they need to consider in order to make a fully informed choice of delivery services. How would you manage this, given that there may be several services competing for the client's care? Also consider the specific issues that older people may have in making these decisions.

C Consumer-directed care is a major component of healthcare within the community setting. How would you, as a care manager, establish policies and practices that would enable your teams to not only understand but also be able to administer this model of practice?

Readings

Pause at this moment and read the following articles. They discuss the philosophies of both consumer-directed and consumer-centred care.

In other words … actively listening for what patients do not say

www.healthliteracy.com/article.asp?PageID=7002

Consumers directing consumer-directed care

www.agedcare.org.au/events-and-conferences/conferences/2012-acsa-national-community-care-conference/presentations-monday-21-may-2012/sue-mckechnie

Person-centred practice

www.health.vic.gov.au/older/toolkit/02PersonCentredPractice/docs/Guide%20to%20implentating%20Person%20centred%20practice.pdf

Patient and consumer centred care

http://www.safetyandquality.gov.au/our-work/patient-and-consumer-centred-care/

Person-centred healthcare

www.mednwh.unimelb.edu.au/pchc/pchc.htm

Health matters: consumer-directed care

www.youtube.com/watch?v=9DLe1ulblbk&hd=1

Inquiry

In their stories, Leonie and Judy both stress the importance of bringing care back to the basics. Leonie stresses a number of times the importance of getting basic nutrition correct, suggesting that we need to 'promote more use of fresh vegetables'. She also says that we should encourage older people to drink more water as it will generally make them feel better within themselves. Judy mentions a number of times the importance of 'considering constipation or medications that they may be on' when treating delirium. She even states: 'I've actually found full resolution of symptoms of delirium simply by treating the constipation or in some cases managing the pain with Panadol'.

As healthcare is becoming increasingly more technical in application, is it possible that we are in danger of neglecting the simple basics of giving care? Judy describes in her case study how a patient who had become agitated at night was calmed simply by turning on the light and spending time with her, although other staff members wanted to administer medications. There was nothing complex about Judy's care. Leonie's speaks about a relative who was exhibiting signs of confusion. These signs soon disappeared once he had simply been given fluids. It was a simple return to considering the basic and unique needs of the patient.

As you listened to Leonie story, you would have heard how the older person is increasingly coming to see her as a client. Where once this would have seemed quite radical, increasing numbers of people are starting to embrace complementary therapies. They do this to not only help maintain their health, but also to assist them when they do have a health compromise. Complementary therapies are based more on traditional approaches to health rather than subscribing to rigorous scientific theory. Some of these traditional approaches may seem familiar to older people.

According to Victoria's Better Health Channel website, the underpinning philosophies of these therapies include an understanding that:

- illness occurs if the body is out of balance
- the body can heal itself given the right conditions
- the person should be treated holistically rather than just the symptoms
- natural products are preferable to synthetic ones.

These are quite simple philosophies and are grounded in the overall belief that we need to get back to the basics of what keeps us healthy and also to simply look at the person as a whole.

Healthcare professionals need to answer the following questions.

- Are we increasingly using medications and technical care at the expense of non-invasive and simpler care activities?
- Do we turn to pharmacological measures as a first resort as the nurse in Judy's story wanted to do, or do we try the simple basics of care first?

Action

A What are the basics, or fundamentals, of care that we offer as healthcare providers? Are these often devalued as unskilled work?

B Given that delirium can be exacerbated or caused by a basic physiological condition, how would you undertake assessment for these conditions prior to

managing delirium as a condition on its own? Who would you involve to assist you?

C How would you develop policy within an acute care environment that clearly sets out the need to consider and undertake the basic fundamentals of care before embarking on a more pharmacological and/or technical approach to care? How would you develop policy that included the use of complementary therapies?

Readings

Review the following articles and think about what they mean for caring practices.

Nursing around

http://nursingaround.blogspot.com.au/2007/12/back-to-basics.html

Technology, health and healthcare

www.health.gov.au/internet/main/publishing.nsf/Content/DA8177ED1A80D332CA257BF0001B08EE/$File/ocpahfsv5.pdf

Why basic nursing care is essential care

www.impactednurse.com/?p=539

Complementary therapies

www.betterhealth.vic.gov.au/bhcv2/bhcarticles.nsf/pages/Complementary_therapies?open

View Polypharmacy, a problem that is easy to ignore

www.youtube.com/watch?v=JY37VcF7EsI&hd=1

A FINAL WORD

Throughout this chapter you have viewed the stories of three individuals, each one considerably different to each other. However, each of our narrators manages to bring to their stories the client's concerns about not being listened to or considered seriously in the management of their care. Clients should always be in control of their own healthcare and treatment. It is their right to be this way as they have a far better knowledge of their body than we do. As health providers, we need to ensure that the client is not only in the centre of the care, but is also informed enough to direct the care that they are to receive.

We also need to ensure that before we plan or manage our care practices, we look carefully at our clients and consider their uniqueness. While we do not wish to negate the importance of using good pharmacological treatments and contemporary technical interventions, we need to think about our client's basic needs first. Although it is at times challenging to us as health professionals to embrace non-traditional mainstream practices, we need to reflect that some of the simple and basic premises of complementary therapies can meet our clients' needs.

By now you should have some insight into caring for your older clients with a health compromise from a basic and holistic perspective and considering their individualities prior to planning and delivering care. There are times when the most simple of care practices, undertaken well, may prevent the use of increased pharmacological and often invasive technical interventions.

CHAPTER 9

Facing Mortality

INTRODUCTION

This chapter consists of two stories with very different perspectives of how a person faces their own mortality and/or that of others around them.

Maureen's is an intimate story. She is a 74-year-old woman who has experienced breast cancer, cared for her mother until her death, cared for her brother and now has her husband living in an aged care facility (ACF). Her story around accepting mortality is very personal and reveals many issues surrounding death and dying.

Shirley is an experienced director of nursing at a residential ACF. Her story focuses on how she actively assists residents and family members to understand and accept their mortality along with the consequences. It is a revealing story and demonstrates how the proactive approaches of health care professionals can assist all involved.

Before you begin ... How perceptions shape the aged care facility experience

Consider the following quote.

> *For most of us, it is almost second nature to defend against the realization of our mortality. Yet each of us has the power to embrace a cultural worldview that gives meaning to life. We can create our own moral compass and build our self-esteem by feeling that we are a valuable member of society. Instead of turning against others, we can use our universal condition as inspiration to treat each other well and to make the most out of the precious time we have.*
> Firestone (2012).

- Do you agree with the above quote?
- Why/why not?
- What are your ideas of mortality?

Many health reports contain mortality rates, used to report the number of deaths due to a certain event such as a disaster or period of time. In this chapter, mortality refers to the realisation that we as people are mortal; we do not live forever. People recognise this at different times of their life and sometimes more than once. Often the death of someone close will initiate thoughts of human mortality; for others it may be a reflection on their life up to a point in time. Some individuals choose to acknowledge and move on while others may start to fear the impending end of their life. Spirituality and religion may become very important to those who consider the idea of their own mortality.

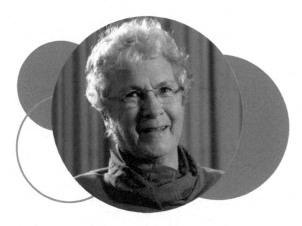

Maureen's story

 View Maureen's story or read the transcript.

Reflection

1. How do you think Maureen adjusted to the changing roles she refers to in the video: having been responsible for the care of everyone else and then having to be a person needing care and attention due to her breast cancer?

2. How does Maureen's perspective of being aware of the 'things of life' assist in her positive outlook on getting older? Does this help you at all? How could others use it?

3. Maureen mentions how she has had the paperwork for the advanced health directive for some time but eventually her daughters had to assist in completing it. Why do you think this was the case?

Inquiry

1. Maureen mentions that she has no fear of death. How do you think previous experiences influence a person's perspective of mortality? What about a person's culture?

2. There are many resources available to help healthcare workers understand various beliefs around facing death. Some examples are found at the following websites.

   http://lmrpcc.org.au/admin/wp-content/uploads/2011/07/Customs-Beliefs-Death-Dying.pdf

   www.health.qld.gov.au/multicultural/health_workers/cultdiver_guide.asp

   www.mcnz.org.nz/assets/News-and-Publications/Statements/best-health-maoricomplete.pdf

a. Access one of these links (or another one of your choice) and examine one culture with which you are not currently familiar.

b. Reflect on how you can assist a person from that culture in continuing to enjoy life despite their ageing years or diagnosis of a terminal illness.

Action

A Describe how important it is to be aware of a person's previous experience with ageing and death. How might you ensure that you translate this awareness into your day-to-day care practice?

B Review your reflections above and relate this to the aged care/clinical setting in which you are either currently employed or have attended on clinical placement. How would this setting provide sensitivity to facing the mortality of a loved one? Are improvements required? If so, what sort of improvements?

C Advanced health directives are an important source of data in ensuring that the person who is facing end-of-life decision making has their views heard and respected. Investigate the role and process of advanced health directives in your work/placement area for your state. How would you, as a healthcare provider, introduce this tool to the family and the person in a respectful manner? Are there instances when it would be inappropriate to do so? How would you manage the situation if the family did not want the person facing death to know about the closeness of their situation and as such not have the opportunity to voice their wishes for their care?

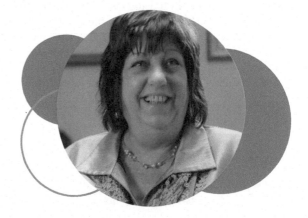

Shirley's story

As mentioned in the introduction, Shirley provides insight as the director of nursing of an ACF on how she and the facility actively assist residents and family members to understand mortality.

 View Shirley's story or read the transcript.

Reflection

1. Shirley has offered some insights into the philosophy of care within an ACF that assist the person to face mortality. What did Shirley consider the most important aspects when caring for an older person and their family?

2. How do you think that fits with current concepts of workloads within an ACF?

3. How can you help ensure that hope is not lost in an older person or their family, regardless of their medical conditions?

4. As mentioned in Shirley's story, 'we are not the judges' when referring to staff outlooks on family members who may choose not to visit their loved one in the ACF. How would you react to a person who does not receive many visits from their family?

Inquiry

Shirley uses the term 'death by inches' when referring to family members who care for a person with dementia. As mentioned elsewhere in this book, a person with dementia has a gradual deterioration of mental functioning and abilities. For those who are close to the person, they slowly lose the person that they know and care for. The person's attitudes, language, behaviours, skills and abilities will often slowly deteriorate and change. Although there are times when the person seems to be the same as they were before their diagnosis of dementia, increasingly these times diminish. It is frequently a long, slow process and family members who observe this often

say they feel as though they are losing this person one bit at a time. This is what Shirley means by 'death by inches'.

1. What do you think of this term? Do you agree or disagree with it?

2. Most people who care for someone with dementia have already experienced a sense of loss, sometimes over a period of up to five years prior to the admission of their loved one into an ACF. Think about how you can assist a family member of someone with dementia who is deteriorating in condition. (Hint: It is *not* to tell them it will be a relief for them and they can then get on with living their lives; the family member is part of their life.)

Action

A Describe how you can encourage the ageing person to maintain a positive outlook on life, regardless of their age. What are some of the more practical things you can do? How would you support them from a psychosocial perspective?

B Review your thoughts on caring for a person with dementia. Often we, as the health care professional, have never had the opportunity to know the person before they developed dementia. How can we ensure that their wishes for end-of-life care are considered?

C As a health care professional, working with the older person will frequently place you in a position of witnessing death and dying. How we manage this is important not just for ourselves, but also for those we care for. How would you, or do you, manage this? What policies and processes will you put into place to ensure that all staff have the opportunity to explore their feelings and beliefs about death and dying? How can you ensure staff who have been involved in the death or palliative care of a person who is near death is coping?

A FINAL WORD

The stories in this chapter have discussed the experiences of older people facing mortality. Understanding these as both a consumer and a manager/health professional provides insights that would be difficult to otherwise gain. The journey to death, and the dying process, is unique to the individual and needs to be considered from a personal perspective. This is one area of health care practice where our thoughts and feelings will impact considerably upon the client's experience. Therefore, it is essential that we care for ourselves in order to give our clients excellent care.

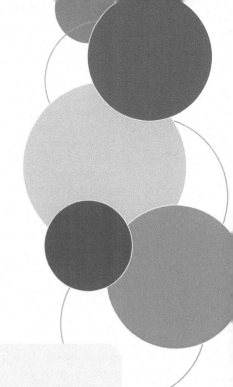

CHAPTER 10

Aged Care Facilities

INTRODUCTION

This chapter consists of two stories that offer very different perspectives surrounding aged care facilities (ACFs). Maureen is a 74-year-old woman whose husband was admitted into an ACF for permanent care 3 years ago. She reveals the issues for her, her husband and at times her family during her story. Shirley is an experienced director of nursing of an ACF so her story focuses on how she perceives the services provided by the facility including challenges for staff, residents and their families.

Before you begin ... Perceptions of aged care facilities

ACFs in Australia were previously known as 'nursing homes', 'aged care hostels' or 'old folks' homes', and many people still use these terms today. In New Zealand they are commonly referred to as 'rest homes'. Reflect on what you think about when you hear these terms.

- Are your thoughts positive or negative?
- Where do you get your perceptions?
- How accurate do you think they are?
- How do you think an older person would feel about these terms? Why?

Aged care facilities

Society's perceptions are often one of the elderly being in either nursing homes or retirement villages, however it must be highlighted that 92% of people over the age of 65 years live in the community, in their home.
(AIHW, 2009)

When health needs necessitate extensive or full-time supervision and care, a long-term care ACF may be the best living option. In Australia there are generally three types of ACFs. These are low-care facilities (previously known as hostels) where the person is partially independent and overall needs supervision or minor assistance with activities of daily living (ADLs) such as showering. There are high-care facilities (previously known as nursing homes) that offer a higher level of care; and there are dementia-specific units, usually with the ability to remain secure so the person can move about freely in the facility but not experience safety issues they may encounter if they could wander freely on roads, for instance. There is also a concept of 'ageing in place', which is designed to allow all residents to continue receiving appropriate care in the ACF as they age, even if this involves a deterioration in their condition since admission. At the time of publication, changes being made to the guidelines for aged care in Australia indicate that the names of these levels of care will no longer be used. This is due to the emphasis of ageing in place, thereby assuming that all levels of care can be provided within the one unit. Despite this the concepts of these levels will continue, particularly at an operational level where factors such as staffing levels and access need to be considered. In all types of facilities, staff are available 24 hours a day with a variety of services to support the medical, personal and psychosocial needs of the ageing client. In New Zealand, while aged care is starting to shift away from previous models, they are currently made up predominantly of rest homes, hospital-funded beds and dementia beds.

At 30 June 2011, in Australia 70% of permanent residents in ACFs were female. Of all female residents, 63% were aged 85 and over, compared with 43% of their male counterparts. Male residents generally had a younger age profile than female residents with 7% entering residential aged care at age 65 or under compared with 2.5% of females (AIHW 2012, p 22).

The majority (74%) of residents admitted to permanent care in 2010–11 were aged 80 and over. The most common age group was 85 to 89, accounting for 29% of permanent admissions, indicating an increase in the number of ageing people within the general population which has consequences for ACFs. It also highlights that people are remaining at home until a much later age than 65 years.

Due to the current admission criteria and processes within the ACFs, it is highly unlikely that if one person from a married couple was admitted into an ACF the other person from that couple would follow; rather, in the majority of cases they would be physically separated as one person lives in the ACF and the other in their home in the community.

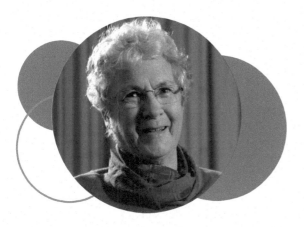

Maureen's story

Begin viewing Maureen's story to 'Bloom where you are planted' or read the transcript.

Maureen refers to her need to change her perspectives as she moves from providing support to her partner to becoming a carer again (as she did when she had a young family) as her husband required more care at home.

Reflection

1. In your plans for the future, do you envisage taking on a role of carer when you are 70 or 80 years old?

2. How do you think life changed for Maureen as she took on a role of carer again?

3. List some examples of how day-to-day planning would change for someone who was initially part of an independent married couple to now becoming a carer for their spouse. How would you react if you suddenly had to care for someone in your family right now?

4. Maureen describes the difficulty she had letting go as a carer and the difficulty she felt not continuing in her carer role after her husband was admitted into the ACF.

5. How do you think you would feel if you had handed over a close family member or even close friend for someone else to now look after?

6. Maureen felt more relaxed when she realised she could visit her husband as his wife, not as his carer. What do you think she meant by this?

7. What do you think would be some of the challenges to her in doing this?

Inquiry

There are many articles that talk about the burden of caring for a loved one as well as the difficulty in making the decision to admit a family member into an ACF with feelings of significant guilt and loss. This can be complicated for a married couple when one person from the couple is admitted to an ACF and is separated from their spouse. Not only does the admission affect the person who was admitted, but it has a major effect on the person who remains at home separated from their spouse.

Search for an article on this topic and summarise the issues it identifies. How do you think you would feel in the position of someone who was going to have a family member admitted to an ACF?

Keeping in the loop

A major issue for those admitted into an ACF is the potential for isolation. This can also be said for the person they have been separated from at home.

Finish viewing Maureen's story or read the transcript.

Maureen discusses the assistance she felt from her family as 'a trouble shared' when dealing with the issues she faced after her husband's admission into the ACF. She also discusses the 6 pm appointment she has every day with him where she sits at home with her glass of wine and waits for the phone to ring. This will be her husband ringing to chat about the day. Maureen mentions the importance of 'keeping him in the loop' but admits she doesn't tell him everything.

Reflection

1. Do you ever share your concerns with a person close to you? How do you feel if they are not available at the time?

2. How would you encourage an older person to share their concerns with others?

3. Why does Maureen choose to not tell her husband everything?

4. What can you do to ensure Maureen maintains a social and active lifestyle, even with her husband residing in an ACF?

Action

A Describe how important it is to maintain family connections and traditions for a person in an ACF. How might you ensure that you translate this awareness into your day-to-day care practice?

B Review your reflections above and relate this to the aged care/clinical setting in which you are either currently employed or have attended on clinical placement. How does this setting encourage the continued connections between the resident in the facility and their family? Do you think this is sufficient?

C Critically review current literature in relation to maintaining social connections for people residing in ACFs. Consider how well this literature informs current practice. Review your organisational policies and procedures in relation to potential barriers that could create difficulty in providing optimum care in this area. Highlight where improvements can be made.

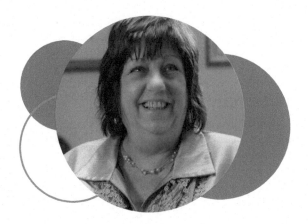

Shirley's story

 Begin viewing Shirley's story to 'Normalisation' or read the transcript.

As mentioned in the introduction and in Chapter 9, Shirley is the director of nursing and manager of an ACF. The ACF consists of high care and low care, including ageing in place and dementia-specific areas. She provides a personal account of her philosophy of care for the residents within the ACF.

Reflection

Shirley offered insights as to what she looks for in a potential staff member applying to work at her ACF.

1. What do you think she means by 'I can train, I can't change values'?

2. How do you think you would fit into her philosophy of staff requirements?

Inquiry

Shirley discusses the power in relationships within the ACF. Access an article about person-centred care and examine it for details of where control is focused between the resident/client and the staff member. Identify the values that are important for ensuring this concept is practised effectively.

Action

A Describe how you would make sure work you were allocated for your shift could be completed while ensuring personal preferences of the resident were considered.

B Explore person-centred care. How can you ensure all staff are able to work to this concept?

C Consider the role of the manager to encourage person-centred care in day-to-day practice within an ACF through policies, procedures and outputs. What outputs could be measured?

Normalisation

When referring to normalisation, it is aimed at the resident (particularly one with dementia) to live in *their* reality.

 Finish viewing Shirley's story or read the transcript.

Reflection

1. How is this different to your expectations of dealing with someone who is confused?
2. How does the person with dementia benefit from this concept?
3. Why is family involvement so important? Who benefits from this involvement?

Inquiry

Access the website below that looks at a village in Norway specifically built to accommodate people with dementia.

Hogewey 'dementia village': the future of dementia care?

http://alz-caregiver.com/hogewey-dementia-village-the-future-of-dementia-care/

Examine the concepts within this village and consider how you could transfer these into an ACF that does not have a physical village in place.

Action

A Describe how your views may have changed about ACFs. Include how you can operate as a staff member in a facility that promotes person-centred care and family involvement.

B Explore the current perceptions in your local community of ACFs. Develop a plan to promote engagement between the local community and ACFs in your area.

C Consider the current funding policies for ACFs. Identify strengths and weaknesses where it supports the ACF to provide person-centred care and strong family involvement. Make recommendations for further consolidation of these areas within ACFs.

A FINAL WORD

This chapter's stories from a consumer and manager/health professional within residential ACFs provide essential insights that would be difficult to gain otherwise. It provides you with insight into how innovation and positive practices can be implemented in the care of those living in ACFs as well as how these can positively impact the family and friends who are also involved in this. Attitude plays an important role and you have been privileged to see it from very personal perspectives. We hope you have enjoyed the experience and that the stories they have so kindly provided will assist you in providing holistic person-centred care to those associated with ACFs.

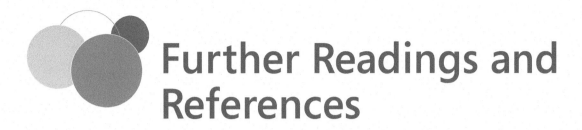

Further Readings and References

Chapter 1

Bowling A, Iliffe S 2011 Psychological approach to successful ageing predicts future quality of life in older adults. Health and Quality of Life Outcomes, 9(13). Available at: www.hqlo.com/content/9/1/13

Harris S, 2011 Do not let them know you are old. Research Magazine, Virginia Tech. Available at: www.research.vt.edu/resmag/2011winter/old.html

Rose MR, Flatt T, Graves JL, Greer LF, Martinez DE, Matos M, Mueller LD, Shmookler Reis RJ, Shahrestani P 2012 What is aging? Frontiers in Genetics. Available at: www.ncbi.nlm.nih.gov/pmc/articles/PMC3400891/

WEBSITES

Aging—Measuring Human Aging: http://medicine.jrank.org/pages/72/Aging-Measuring-human-aging.html

COTA for older Australians: www.cota.org.au/australia/

ElderWeb: www.elderweb.com

My Aged Care: www.myagedcare.gov.au

Older Aboriginal and Torres Strait Islander people: www.aihw.gov.au/publication-detail/?id=10737418972 www.aihw.gov.au/indigenous-observatory-older-people/

Summary of ageing among indigenous people: www.healthinfonet.ecu.edu.au/health-facts/health-faqs/aboriginal-population

What do we know about the ageing population: http://www.healthinfonet.ecu.edu.au/population-groups/older-people/reviews/our-review

Chapter 2

Giles LC, Glonek GFV, Luszcz MA & Andrews GR 2005 Effect of social networks on 10 year survival in very old Australians: the Australian longitudinal study of aging. Journal of Epidemiology and Community Health 59(7):574–579. Available at: http://jech.bmj.com/content/59/7/574.short

McLaughlin D, Vagenas D, Pachana NA, Begum N, Dobson A 2010 Gender differences in social network size and satisfaction in adults in their 70s. Journal of Health Psychology 15(5):671–679. Available at: www.ncbi.nlm.nih.gov/pubmed/20603290

Seth Cohen A 2012 Advanced Style. Powerhouse Books, US

Steptoe A, Shankar A, Demakakos P, Wardle J 2013 Social isolation, loneliness, and all-cause mortality in older men and women. Proceedings of National Academy of Science 110 (15):5797–5801. Available at: www.pnas.org/content/110/15/5797

WEBSITES

Probus Association of Queensland: www.paqnetwork.asn.au

Quota International: www.quota.org/about-quota/

Soroptimist International: www.soroptimistinternational.org

Toastmasters International: www.toastmasters.org

Volunteering Queensland: http://volunteeringqld.org.au/web/

Chapter 3

Australian Bureau of Statistics 2009 Experimental life tables for Aboriginal and Torres Strait Islanders Australia 2005–2007 Cat no. 3302.0.55.003. ABS, Canberra

Australian Indigenous Health InfoNet 2012 Overview of Australian Indigenous health status. Available at: www.healthinfonet.ecu.edu.au

Dance P, Brown R, Bammer G, Sibthorpe B 2004 Aged care services for indigenous people in the Australian Capital Territory and surrounds: analysing needs and implementing change. Australian and New Zealand Journal of Public Health 28(6):379–383

MacRae A, Thomson N, Anomie, Burns J, Catto M, Gray C, Levitan L, McLoughlin N, Potter C, Ride K, Stumpers S, Trzesinski A, Urquhart B 2013 Overview of Australian Indigenous health status, 2012. Available at: www.healthinfonet.ecu.edu.au

Singh P, Hussain R, Khan A, Irwin L, Foskey R 2014 Dementia care: intersecting informal family care and formal care systems. Journal of Aging Research. Available at: www.hindawi.com/journals/jar/2014/486521/

SCRGSP (Steering Committee for the Review of Government Service Provision) 2011 Overcoming Indigenous Disadvantage: Key Indicators 2011, Productivity Commission, Canberra. Available at: www.pc.gov.au/gsp/overcoming-indigenous-disadvantage/key-indicators-2011

Silverstein M, Giarrusso R 2010 Aging and family life: a decade review. Journal of Marriage and Family 72(5):1039–1058.

WEBSITES

Fred Hollows Foundation: www.hollows.org.au/our-work/australia

National Aboriginal Community Controlled Health Organisation: www.naccho.org.au

Chapter 4

Australian Population and Migration Research Centre (APMRC) September 2013 FEECA Systematic review: a systemic review of Australian research on older people from CALD background to provide and promote translation of research into CALD aged practices: discussion paper. Initially prepared by Dr Kelly McDougall & Dr Helen Feist, Australian Population and Migration Research Centre (APMRC). School of Social Sciences, University of Adelaide SA. Available at: www.adelaide.edu.au/apmrc

Department of Health. The community-based aged care workforce—a desktop review of the literature January 2006: culturally and linguistically diverse (CALD) communities—related information: www.health.gov.au/internet/publications/publishing.nsf/Content/ageing-twf-cbw-lit-review~ageing-twf-cbw-lit-review-ATSI-CALD~ageing-twf-cbw-lit-review-CALD

Social Policy Research Centre and The Benevolent Society October 2010 Supporting older people from culturally diverse backgrounds. Research to Practice Briefing 4. The Benevolent Society. Available at: https://www.sprc.unsw.edu.au/media/SPRCFile/10_Report_BenSoc_ResearchtoPractice4.pdf

Warburton J, McLaughlin D 2007 Passing on our culture: how older Australians from diverse cultural backgrounds contribute to civil society. Journal of Cross-Cultural Gerontology 22(1):47–60. Available at: http://link.springer.com/article/10.1007/s10823-006-9012-4

WEBSITES

Centre for Cultural Diversity in Ageing: www.culturaldiversity.com.au

Diversicare: http://diversicare.com.au

Multicultural Aged Care Inc.: www.mac.org.au

Chapter 5

Bouman WP, Arcelus J, Benbow SM 2006 Nottingham study of sexuality & ageing (NoSSA I). Attitudes regarding sexuality and older people: a review of the literature. Sexual and Relationship Therapy 21(2):149–161. Available at: www.tandfonline.com/doi/abs/10.1080/14681990600618879#.UszT80l-_mQ

Bouman WP, Arcelus J, Benbow SM 2007 Nottingham study of sexuality and ageing (NoSSA II). Attitudes of care staff regarding sexuality and residents: A study in residential and nursing homes. Sexual and Relationship Therapy 22(1):45–61. Available at: www.tandfonline.com/doi/abs/10.1080/14681990600637630#.UszTsUl-_mQ

Department of Health 20 December 2012 National Lesbian, Gay, Bisexual, Transgender and Intersex (LGBTI) Ageing and Aged Care Strategy. Available at: www.health.gov.au/internet/main/publishing.nsf/Content/ageing-lgbti-national-aged-care-strategy-html

Elias J, Ryan A 2011 A review and commentary on the factors that influence expressions of sexuality by older people in care homes. Journal of Clinical Nursing 20(11–12):1668–1676. Available at: http://onlinelibrary.wiley.com/doi/10.1111/j.1365-2702.2010.03409.x/abstract

Hayward LE, Robertson N, Knight C 2013 Inappropriate sexual behaviour and dementia: An exploration of staff experiences. Dementia 12(4):463–480. Available at: http://dem.sagepub.com/content/12/4/463.abstract

Lindau ST, Schumm LP, Edward MA, Laumann O, Levinson W, O'Muircheartaigh CA, Waite LJ Aug 2007 A study of sexuality and health among older adults in the United States. New England Journal of Medicine 357:762–774. Available at: www.nejm.org/doi/full/10.1056/NEJMoa067423

Queensland Dementia Training Study Centres 9 May 2013 Sexualities and Dementia: Education Resource for Health Professionals. Available at: www.dtsc.com.au/sexualities-and-dementia-8-5-2013

Queensland Law Reform Commission September 2008 Shaping Queensland's guardianship legislation: principles and capacity, discussion paper WP No. 64. Available at: http://www.qlrc.qld.gov.au/wpapers/wp64.pdf

Short M 27 June 2011 Joan McCarthy is turning accepted notions of ageing and sexuality on their head. Sydney Morning Herald. Available at: www.smh.com.au/federal-politics/society-and-culture/the-time-of-her-life-20110626-1gllx.html

Smith D 26 June 2013 Discrimination against older LGBTI people should be addressed by new law. The Guardian. Available at www.guardian.co.uk/commentisfree/2013/jun/26/older-lgbti-people-discrimination-law

Ward R, Vass AA, Aggarwal N, Garfield C, Cybyk B 2005 A kiss is still a kiss? The construction of sexuality in dementia care. Dementia 4(1):49–72. Available at: http://dem.sagepub.com/content/4/1/49.short

WEBSITES

Australian Law Reform Commission: www.alrc.gov.au

Department of Health and Ageing: www.dss.gov.au/our-responsibilities/ageing-and-aged-care/aged-care-reform

LGBT Ageing Action Group: Healthy Communities, along with other organisations including the Gay & Lesbian Welfare Association and the Commonwealth Respite and Carelink Centre have formed an LGBT Ageing Action Group: www.qahc.org.au/ageing

LGBTI Seniors—Lesbian, Gay, Bisexual and Transgender Ageing & Seniors' Items of Interest (Linking Seniors with Community Information): www.seniorsenquiryline.com.au

Chapter 6

Broderick E 2013 Caring for the carers. The Australian. Available at: www.theaustralian.com.au/national-affairs/opinion/caring-for-the-carers/story-e6frgd0x-1226585430408#

Carer Recognition Act 2010 (Cwlth). Available at: www.comlaw.gov.au/Details/C2010A00123

Carers Australia May 2008 Submission to the National Health and Hospitals Reform Commission. Available at: www.health.gov.au/internet/nhhrc/publishing.nsf/Content/055-ca/$FILE/Submissions%20055%20-%20Carers%20Australia%20Submission.pdf

Carers Australia July 2010 Submission to the Productivity Commission Inquiry into Caring for Older Australians. Available at: www.carersaustralia.com.au/storage/Submission to PC Caring Older Australians.pdf

Carers Australia 28 September 2012 Carers caught in the 'sandwich generation'. Available at: www.carersaustralia.com.au/media-centre/article/?id=carers-caught-in-the-sandwich-generation

Caring for yourself while caring for others: fact sheet. Available at: https://au.reachout.com/Factsheets/C/Caring-for-yourself-while-caring-for-others#other

Diller V October 3 2012 The 'Over-Stuffed' sandwich generation. Psychology Today. Available at: www.psychologytoday.com/blog/face-it/201210/the-over-stuffed-sandwich-generation

Grundy E, Henretta J 2006 Between elderly parents and adult children: a new look at the intergenerational care provided by the 'sandwich generation'. Ageing and Society 26:707–722. Available at: http://journals.cambridge.org/action/displayFulltext?type=1&fid=458803&jid=ASO&volumeId=26&issueId=05&aid=458802&bodyId=&membershipNumber=&societyETOCSession=

Kingsmill S, Schlesinger B 1998 The family squeeze: surviving the sandwich generation. University of Toronto, Canada. Available at: http://books.google.com.au/books?hl=en&lr=&id=eOx0hkn4i1AC&oi=fnd&pg=PR9&dq=the+sandwich+generation&ots=O8lotMu1p0&sig=gWmDZXJwepUgj0yUC6hJ9H65ksc#v=onepage&q=the%20sandwich%20generation&f=false

Kunemund H 2006 Changing welfare states and the 'sandwich generation': increasing burden for the next generation? International Journal of Ageing and Later Life 1(2). Available at: www.ep.liu.se/ej/ijal/2006/v1/i2/ijal06v1i2b-complete_issue.pdf#page=11

Mascarella J n.d. Meet the sandwich generation. Parenting. Available at: www.parenting.com/article/sandwich-generation

Monin JK, Schultz R September 2009 Interpersonal effects of suffering in older adult caregiving relationships. Psychology and Aging, 24(3):681–695.

Neuhausen C 29 April 2010 The sandwich generation: baby boomers feel the squeeze. Pasadena Weekly. Available at: www.pasadenaweekly.com/cms/story/detail/the_sandwich_generation/8694/

Power, J 28 July 2012 The sandwich generation. Sydney Morning Herald. Available at: www.smh.com.au/national/the-sandwich-generation-20120727-22zj2.html

Raphael D, Schlesinger B 1994 Women in the sandwich generation: do adult children living at home help? Journal of Women and Aging 6:21–45.

Snow K, Naaman L 20 March 2008 Sandwich generation faces massive stress in caring for aging parents and kids. Available at: http://abcnews.go.com/GMA/Parenting/story?id=4487229

Stritof S, Stritof R n.d. The sandwich generation: the cluttered nest syndrome. Available at: http://marriage.about.com/cs/sandwich/a/sandwichgen.htm

The sandwich generation: caring for kids and your parents. Available at: www.agingcare.com/Articles/The-Sandwich-Generation-caring-for-Children-and-elderly-parents-123286.htm

Williams C September 2004 The sandwich generation perspectives on labour and income. Statistics Canada 5(9). Available at: www.statcan.gc.ca/pub/75-001-x/10904/7033-eng.htm

Wintz S The Sandwich generation. Available at: www.summitplanninggrp.com/files/34865/Market%20Update%20From%20Summit%20Planning%20Group%20May%202010.pdf

Zal HM 2009 The sandwich generation: caught between growing children and aging parents. Perseus, Massachusetts.

WEBSITES

Care Giver Stress: www.caregiverstress.com/stress-management/

Carer Allowance: http://www.humanservices.gov.au/customer/services/centrelink/carer-allowance

Carers Australia: www.carersaustralia.com.au

Department of Human Services: www.humanservices.gov.au

Health Direct Australia: www.healthdirect.gov.au

My Aged Care: www.myagedcare.gov.au/caring-someone/counselling-and-support-carers

Old Mutual Savings Monitor:
http://160.123.226.43/documents/SavingsMonitor/SandwichGeneration_November2010.pdf

Parenting: www.parenting.com

Respite care: www.healthdirect.gov.au

The Sandwich Generation: www.sandwichgeneration.com

Chapter 7

Daskein R, Moyle W, Creedy D 2009 Aged-care nurses' knowledge of nursing documentation: an Australian perspective. Journal of Clinical Nursing 18(14):2087–2095

Queensland Law Reform Commission September 2008 Shaping Queensland's guardianship legislation: principles and capacity, discussion paper WP No. 64. Available at:
http://www.qlrc.qld.gov.au/wpapers/wp64.pdf

Staunton P, Chiarella M 2012 Law for Nurses and Midwives, 7th edn. Churchill Livingstone, Australia.

WEBSITES

Aged Care Act 1997 (Cwlth): www.comlaw.gov.au/Details/C2014C00316

Department of Health and Ageing:
www.dss.gov.au/our-responsibilities/ageing-and-aged-care/aged-care-reform

Information Privacy Act 2009 (Qld):
www.qld.gov.au/law/your-rights/privacy-and-right-to-information/privacy-rights

Leading Age Services Australia Queensland (LASA Q): www.qld.lasa.asn.au

My Aged Care: www.myagedcare.gov.au

Chapter 8

Australian Bureau of Statistics 2008 Complementary therapies. Australian Social Trends. cat. no. 4102.0. ABS, Canberra. Available at: www.abs.gov.au/AUSSTATS/abs@.nsf/Lookup/4102.0Chapter5202008

Australian Commission on Safety and Quality in Healthcare. Patient and consumer centred care discussion paper. Available at: www.safetyandquality.gov.au/our-work/patient-and-consumer-centred-care/

Britton ME 2011 Drugs, delirium and older people. Journal of Pharmacy Practice and Research 41(3). Available at: http://jppr.shpa.org.au/lib/pdf/2011_09/Mary_Britton_GT.pdf

Dogget J February 2002 Review of The desktop guide to complementary and alternative medicine: an evidence-based approach. Chest 121(2):670. Available at:
http://journal.publications.chestnet.org/pdfaccess.ashx?ResourceID=2103906&PDFSource=13

Ernst E, Pittler MH, Stevinson C, White A (eds) 2001 The Desktop Guide to Complementary and Alternative Medicine: An Evidence-based Approach. Harcourt Publishers, Ltd., London

HealthWorkforce Australia. Caring for older people program. Available at:
www.hwa.gov.au/our-work/boost-productivity/caring-older-people-program

State Government of Victoria, Department of Health. Person-centred practice. Available at:
www.health.vic.gov.au/older/toolkit/02PersonCentredPractice/index.htm

WEBSITES

Australian Government Department of Human Services:
www.humanservices.gov.au; www.hwa.gov.au/our-work/boost-productivity/caring-older-people-program

Department of Health Services—Older Australians:
www.humanservices.gov.au/customer/themes/older-australians

Health Direct Australia: www.healthdirect.gov.au

My Aged Care: www.myagedcare.gov.au/caring-someone/counselling-and-support-carers

Victorian Government Health Information Person-centred practice:
www.health.vic.gov.au/older/toolkit/02PersonCentredPractice/

Victoria's Better Health Channel:
www.betterhealth.vic.gov.au/bhcv2/bhcarticles.nsf/pages/Complementary_therapies?open

Chapter 9

Clark K, Philips J April 2010 End of life care: the importance of culture and ethnicity. Australian Family Physician 39(4). Available at: www.ncbi.nlm.nih.gov/pubmed/20372679

Firestone L 2012 Creating meaning by facing our mortality: how death awareness can help us make conscious choices to live more fully. Compassion Matters. Available at:
www.psychologytoday.com/blog/compassion-matters/201205/creating-meaning-facing-our-mortality

MacLeod R, Vella-Brincat J, Macleod A 2012 The Palliative Care Handbook: Guidelines For Clinical Management and Symptom Control, New Zealand. Available at:
www.hospice.org.nz/cms_show_download.php?id=377

WEBSITES

Australian Living Wills Registry: http://auslwr.com.

Centre for Cultural Diversity in Ageing:
www.culturaldiversity.com.au/resources/practice-guides/palliative-care

Ministry of Social Development: https://www.msd.govt.nz/what-we-can-do/seniorcitizens/

My Aged Care: www.myagedcare.gov.au

Palliative Care Australia: www.palliativecare.org.au/Home.aspx

The Life Resources Charitable Trust: www.life.org.nz/euthanasia/euthanasialegalkeyissues/living-wills

Chapter 10

Australian Institute of Health and Welfare 2009. Australia's Welfare 2009. Australia's welfare series no 9 cat. no. AUS 117. AIHW, Canberra

Australian Institute of Health and Welfare 2012 Residential Aged Care in Australia 2010–11: A Statistical Overview. Aged care statistics series 36 cat. no. AGE 68. AIHW, Canberra

Botek A 2012 How different countries infuse dignity into dementia care. Available at:
www.agingcare.com/Articles/different-countries-making-dementia-care-dignified-161973.htm (This website allows you to explore dementia friendly communities thought the world, including Australia.)

Brown L, Nepal B, Thurecht L 2012 Aged care in Australia: past present and future. Available at:
www.natsem.canberra.edu.au/storage/Brown%20-%20Aged%20care%20-%20past%20present%20future.pdf

Hans B 2012 Living in the moment: Dutch village offers dignified care for dementia sufferers. SPIEGEL ONLINE International. Available at:
www.spiegel.de/international/europe/dutch-village-for-elderly-with-dementia-offers-alternative-care-a-824582.html

Schmid C 21 August 2013 Hogewey 'dementia village': the future of dementia care? Available at:
www.best-alzheimers-products.com/hogewey-dementia-village-the-future-of-dementia-care.html

WEBSITES

Aged Care in Victoria: www.health.vic.gov.au/agedcare/services/residential.htm

Australian Institute of Health and Welfare (AIHW) Aged care: www.aihw.gov.au/aged-care/

Department of Health Aged care information:
www.health.gov.au/internet/main/publishing.nsf/Content/ageing-aged-care-information.htm

Ministry of Health New Zealand Residential care questions and answers:
www.health.govt.nz/our-work/life-stages/health-older-people/long-term-residential-care/residential-care-questions-and-answers

My Aged Care: www.myagedcare.gov.au

New Zealand Aged Care Association: http://nzaca.org.nz

Transcripts

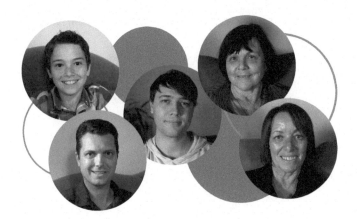

CHAPTER 1

The Panel's story

Lachlan:	Hello, my name is Lachlan. I'm 12 and currently attending primary school.
Theo:	My name is Theo. I'm 26 and I'm a retail manager.
Brendan:	My name is Brendan. I'm 40 and I'm an RF design engineer.
Helen:	I'm Helen. I'm in my 50s and I run a shelter and a council pound facility.

Anne: My name is Anne. I'm 66 and I'm a retired school teacher.

Do you consider yourself old?

Anne: Well, when you say consider yourself old, there's two aspects to look at it: you could either be chronologically or how you feel mentally. Well, I feel I'm approaching old age, because I'm 66 and I think physically old age I would class coming after 70 because of all the physical changes, but mentally everybody is different. And at the moment I still feel I'm enjoying life, and I don't feel incapacitated by my disabilities.

Theo: At work obviously there's a lot of people still at school, so when I compare myself to them I definitely do feel old, but then on the same hand, a lot of the customers that come, they struggle even to get their own groceries or whatnot and then I feel quite young in contrast to them.

Brendan: I wouldn't consider myself old yet, but at the same time I'm becoming more aware of the passage of time. It ranges from things like physically I'm not as fit or as strong as I used to be and also when I compare myself to the younger staff coming through at work, as you have staff leaving and new staff come on board, I'm aware that I don't share the same interests or pastimes as the younger staff, the way they talk, the way they behave, the way they dress, it is subtly different I guess to how people of my age talk and dress.

Lachlan: I don't consider myself old yet, because I'm not a teenager yet, but it depends on different aspects of my life, because at school I'm in grade 7 which means top-of-the-food-chain kind of thing, but anything outside I consider myself really young, because I don't contain the information that other people do.

Helen: Physically I may have slowed down a little bit in the last few years, mentally I've never felt better, I'm a long way off being old.

What age is old?

Theo: A lot of your responsibilities seem to change around your mid- to late 20s and then your 30s. I'd say as the whole of society we start to head towards a new family route at 30; yeah, your responsibilities change and I guess it's more like maturing as opposed to getting old.

Lachlan: 18, the age of, you know, being old, because anything below 18 you don't have any of the responsibilities, so at 18 you get your driver's licence and that's the age you're allowed to work in, but anything really below that, you still rely on a lot of people to feed you or bring money.

Helen: I don't think you can really put an age on old. Like Theo said, some people are old at 30, there's people at 90 years old that really aren't old. I think it all depends on where you are and what stage you are in your life.

Anne: Looking at it physically I agree that you can have a very young outlook, but physically I can't escape the fact that I think about 70, obviously you get some people still marathon runners, but they're few and far between, but I think you're slowing down a bit physically at 70. So from my own point of view I feel I'm 66, I think I'm slowing down a little bit and I think I will slow down even more at 70 onwards, yes.

Brendan: I think if I had to put a number on it I'd probably say somewhere around 70, but I think in general the word 'old' does have a connotation that to me implies increasing physical infirmity, implies increasing dependence on others for your day-to-day welfare and healthcare needs. It implies someone who is not working most of the time, so I think for me the term, when I consider someone to be old is when someone is less independent and less self-sufficient.

What are older people like?

Helen: My mother. Dismal outlook, bad attitude—love my mother, don't get me wrong—but she's got a very old attitude: everything is a problem, physically she's always got 'oh this hurts', 'that hurts', 'oh wish this', 'wish that'—that's an old person.

Theo: An older person, like has been said, can vary; sometimes they look quite decrepit you'd say, can't really do a lot for themselves, but on the other hand I dare say a lot of responsibilities can maybe weigh someone down, take away their freedom and I guess that could class them as old. So I guess anybody who doesn't have, I guess, the freedom to basically do whatever they want.

Brendan: I think it's actually getting harder to tell, because older people these days I think are possibly more fashion conscious than people of their parents' generation. I guess I look at people like my mother and father and they dress quite fashionably: they're quite conscious about having clothing that's reasonably fashionable. Mum's always keeping her hair looking reasonably contemporary and I think older people these days are more health conscious, so their diet, I think, is probably better. Many of them try and quit smoking and cut down on their drinking and exercise more, so there's a lot of people in their 60s and even 70s these days who look fantastic and dress very well. So obviously all the fashion consciousness in the world won't hide the wrinkles and so forth and loss of muscle tone, etc., but it's not always easy to tell how old someone is these days for all of those reasons.

What should older people not do?

Brendan: Something that I think an older person should not do is behave in a way that's not age appropriate, or rather, try and change their behaviour to try and appear to be a member of a younger demographic. So using the sort of slang that younger people would normally use or dressing in a way that, say, a 20 year old would normally dress, I think that kind of thing, I don't think it fools anybody and I think it looks a little undignified to see an older person doing that. If they actually like those fashions or like that music or mode of speech that's fine, but if they're doing it as a way of appearing young and hip, I don't think it's a good look.

Theo: An older person should generally not be the central focus point of anything really, sort of just be there, but not necessarily seen or heard, as terrible as that sounds. Obviously an older person has a lot of experiences, but not I'd say you'd maybe call it the clown or class clown per se, but …

Helen: I don't think they should impose their beliefs of what was right for them and that generation upon what people are doing now without fully understanding it.

Lachlan: I think older people shouldn't use their bodies so aggressively as young people, because if an older person was to damage their body in some way, it would take a much, much longer time to actually heal itself, which means any contact sports, if you fell over and grazed your arm, you might not be able to use it.

Anne: If you're healthy enough, if you can take it, I think you do what you want to do.

What happens as people get older?

Brendan: Something that I have observed about older people is they seem to reach a certain age where they are no longer quite so concerned about what other people think and they increasingly speak and behave in a way to please themselves. And I've noticed that a lot of older people can be quite assertive and quite outspoken in their opinions, that they don't seem to be quite so concerned about offending other people; they don't set out deliberately to offend other people, but they just become forthright, I suppose.

Anne: You think more about death so you think, 'Right. Well, I'm not going to just sit back and be complacent.'

Theo: It's more of a shifting set of responsibilities, sort of changes … your values. Obviously, as you start off younger, your values are obviously lots of materialistic possessions and then as you get older you start to sway away from materialistic possessions and then you turn into more focused on yourself, what you look like and not necessarily just for you, but a lot of you want to portray an image that everybody can see you as. But then once you go on from that you obviously start to develop a family and obviously your own personal image: it's not quite your central focus any more. And it starts towards your family and then obviously your family gets older and they move out and then again maybe you come back to your own self-image, but it isn't you focus on your image for other people to sort of look at and say, 'hey look at me', but it's your own self-image for you.

Lachlan: When a person grows up they kind of wake up to the world and realise that 'I have to fend for myself now', they won't always go to the local club or the bar and party till 12 o'clock because it's the weekend or something, that they have to take it easy for a little bit, because you've got work or you've got to do something.

What makes a person old?

Lachlan: You start obsessing over the little things, like if something comes to you, like a word, you start obsessing what does that word mean, your life starts to revolve around this one thing. And so you kind of have to focus on that all the time and then you can move on after knowing what it is.

Helen: If you think you are old, then you are old. I know people far, far younger than me that think they're old and they really are old people. So I think it's all about your own positive attitude.

Anne: I think a lot of it is to do with your physical health and wellbeing, so I think that's very important.

Theo: I would say the most probably obvious one would be the ability to contribute to society or sustain themselves or I guess the physical thing is probably the most age process. I mean obviously there are the extremes where your mind can probably go before your body but I'd say nine times out of 10 it's definitely physical appearance and abilities.

Brendan: What makes a person old I think is to me it's lack of independence, lack of mobility, also possibly a retreat from the everyday cut and thrust of pop culture and I imagine that by the time you reach, say, the age of 70 or 80 all the political discussions and the political spin that could ever exist you've seen it a hundred times, so you maybe become a bit disconnected from the day-to-day issues. So it's a retreat perhaps from society or from that sort of social conversation.

How would you know when you are old?

Brendan: I think first of all I would know I was old because my kids tell me, 'What would you know, Dad? You're old' so that would be one. I guess what I'm saying is that it's quite natural to measure yourself up against other people or compare yourself to other people and I guess you'll perceive these differences emerging over time. So I guess there's obviously the physical decline as well, which I suppose accumulates over time.

Theo: Compared to some I feel I'm young, compared to some I'm old. I guess the real one is when I feel I no longer can contribute much to society.

Anne: Well, I think it's a very gradual process, like I noticed that I'm going to the doctor's more now for different things. If you're in pain all the time you're bound to have bad depression and things like that, because lots of old people are on antidepressants because of the pain. For older people I think it's when physically you're just deteriorating and if you can't see … like I would dread to lose my eyes, because I like reading and drawing.

What will your generation be like when they are deemed to be old?

Helen: Once again, this is a bit of a tricky question because it depends on, with technology we can still be social and never leave our homes, which means we can enhance our image any way we like, great technologies and surgery: we can all have surgery. I reckon we're going to be a good-looking generation when we get older. I think we're going to look really good.

Lachlan: I think it really depends on the person, because take just people at school: they don't bother to brush their hair before they come to school, brush their teeth or don't do their top button up or something and so I think that would depend on the elderly too. It kind of depends if they want to be seen as looking still in their youth or just 'this is who I am, accept me for who I am' kind of thing.

Anne: If we want to look pretty good we've got the means these days, you can get your hair done, face lifts if you want to.

Theo: There'll be more mobility, obviously there would probably be social media, advancements in technology in terms of electric carts, limb replacement, but in all essence it'll probably just be superseded by the younger generation. So what my generation will have as elders or old people will be great compared to now.

Brendan: My generation still very much is the fast-food generation and also we lead very sedentary lives. Most people these days or very many people that I know they sit in front of a PC all day as their job and I can see these guys that I work with: with every passing month I can see them getting fatter and their shoulders getting rounder and they don't look healthy. And it may be that by the time they start to become more aware of these issues it may be too late for them, so there's competing forces there, our sedentary lives balanced off against the advances in medical technology.

Would you live with your children if you needed care?

Lachlan: If you have to be fed at a specific time and have your afternoon nap then I guess it would be a chore, but if everyone has dinner at the same time, you eat breakfast, lunch, then it feels like you're part of the family and not like a pet, I guess.

Brendan: I think that something else I would also be conscious of, even if there was a sense of welcoming and a loving kind of relationship between me and the child and their spouse, I'd still be conscious of the fact that people these days are living longer and longer. So if I was to move in with them at the age of 70 I could still be with them at the age of 100 when they're approaching old age themselves. And I think that what may start out as a friendly loving environment may become more resentful over time.

Who should be responsible for caring for the older person?

Theo: It's difficult to say … I would say, the family. I don't feel that the government should have to look after elderly people once they're beyond their own living. Obviously as a son I would care for my mother, but like I said the responsibility should fall back on the family, but that again obviously creates a harsh reality where obviously some people just won't have that. And whether or not the government picks up the slack is …

Anne: I think it should be the government, should be very high-quality care, because some families are not an all-loving and they just want you to die so they can get your money and all this kind of thing.

Helen: I really believe the community should care for their older people, you know, the families, the communities and, this is going on experiences once again. We had an old lady that lived up the top of the road from us and as a community we all had our own very, very different roles and we gave that lady very good quality of life. I would like to think that we, as a society we should be providing that to these people that all contributed towards our society, making society what it is. Obviously you'd have to look at government funding, the money would have to come from somewhere, but I think the care should come from the community.

Final comment …

Brendan: As people that I know have gotten older, they've often become more interested in ideas, they've become more spiritual often, not necessarily religious, but certainly much more aware to, I guess, mortality and how to live a good life, what's important in life and so forth. And I guess just very interested in ways of living and ways of having good healthy relationships, that maybe they didn't have time to reflect on these things so much back when they were married with kids and doing the nine-to-five grind. So many older people that I know have become more thoughtful and more interesting as they've grown older.

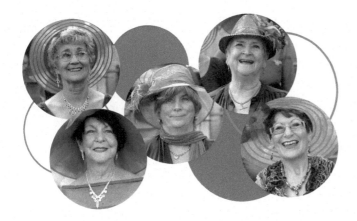

CHAPTER 2

The Red Hat Ladies' story

Positive ageing

Dawn: Hi, my name's Dawn and I'm the queen of Bubbles and butterflies. At the age of 70, I decided to finish work because I had to have time to play. So I've been playing with bubbles and butterflies for 4 years.

Anna: My name's Anna and I'm 67 years old. I've been a Red Hatter for four years. Totally love my red hats, committed to it. The only time I miss is when I'm overseas or family or at work. Still working, totally love my job. Everything I do in life now, I do for fun and friendship. And I'm really at a good place.

Sandy: My name's Sandy. I've been a Red Hatter for five years. I've been with Dawn since she started her chapter. My name is Lady Dilligaf. I have joined the Red Hats to have a bit of fun in my life and that I do.

Lorna: My name's Lorna. My chapter name is Lady Lorna. I'm in my early seventies. I joined Red Hats about 6 months ago. And I joined it because it's a fun thing and it's not a fundraising thing. I'm a delegate for View Clubs of Australia and that's a big job and a responsible job. So I enjoy that but I enjoy Red Hats for different reasons. I've got three grown-up children and my husband lives in a different country so we see each other about every 2 months. So I'm a part-time wife. Apart from that, I have no responsibilities to anybody and I thoroughly enjoy that. In my life I've had very responsible jobs. I was a nursing university tutor for many years and was glad to get out of that. The politics were a bit too … got a bit too much. But I did enjoy that and it was great. But I'm enjoying this phase of my life very, very much.

Carol: Hi, my name is Carol. I spend a bit of time travelling around Australia which I really enjoy. I'm 67 and retired with a lot of responsibilities and doing various charitable things. So I wanted some time for myself and I wanted to make some new friends and just have a great time, as I was getting older, growing up, yeah. Red Hats is just a great way of doing it. They're just a great bunch of ladies and we have a good time.

Bubbles and butterflies—learning to have fun!

Dawn: Well, I was discussing names with my daughter when I decided to start a chapter. And Tania's 50, a very young 50. And we travel together and get on like sisters, she's my very best friend. And we thought well, she said she doesn't drink but I love bubbles. So we called it 'bubbles', and 'butterflies' are for flitting around and having fun. And that's exactly what the group does. And even though we've all got different issues in our life, when we're together, we don't talk about being sick. We talk about what can we do next. Little Anna over here at the weekend away, danced like she was a 15 year old and had a blast. And she doesn't even drink the bubbles.

Importance of being part of a group

Lorna: When I joined this group, the first thing that Dawn said, 'well you've got to make your own hat'. My god! Make my own hat? And I came here making hats and Dawn helped me make a hat. And to me, that was something really, really different. It makes you extend. It's not a group that's banging a drum for something; I'm already a member of one of those. It's just relaxing and it's just great. And we laugh a lot, and, we had a lovely lunch yesterday and it's just lovely.

Making the most of every day

Anna: I think we're all most grateful for being healthy. And because we enjoy good health, we make the most of every day as it comes along. And try and make all our people around us also feel the happiness.

Carol: I think probably all of us have got lots and lots of responsibilities, but haven't had time to nurture other friendships and this was a good way of starting. We're only young.

Outings, friendships and fun

Anna: We have lots of dinners out, lunches, breakfasts. In fact, sometimes I think I should join a club that doesn't involve eating, like a book club or a walking club … but all this eating! But hey, that's good too. But we go to shows and I'm sure a few of you get together and you might go to movies or even just walks. And it's the outings as well as the friendship and the fun.

Carol: And the dressing up.

Anna: That's exactly right, the dressing up.

Carol: It's a good opportunity to dress up and put your makeup on.

Lorna: And we can laugh together. And people look at us and think, 'they're having a good time'. But I mean, they probably wonder what the hell you thought you were playing at walking down the street looking like that.

Dawn: Well, they stop you and ask and then a lot of them want to join you, don't they? Yeah, it's great.

Leaving everything else behind

Sandy: With the Red Hats, it's a time to have fun and leave all ailments behind. Leave everything else behind and enjoy life.

Carol: It's a time of our life to enjoy and do the things that perhaps we've wanted to and haven't had the time to do. And just go out there and try something different.

Pushing the boundaries

Sandy: They push the boundaries sometimes and get you out there doing things that you would not normally do. And for that, I've just really appreciated it and I will be a Red Hatter for life.

Carol: The only groups that I've ever been in from a young girl right up until now have always been centred around fundraising for some organisation or charity or whatever. And this is the first time I've been in an organisation that's all about the girls. Not what you can do for somebody else. And I think that's important because women generally are responsible for a lot of other people.

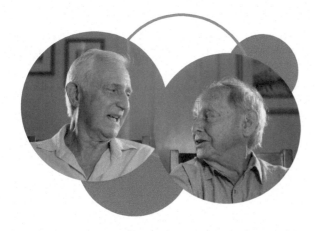

CHAPTER 2

Ron and Larry's story

Introducing Ron

Ron: I'm Ron Prescott. I'm just 80 years young this month and we are English of heritage, we came to Australia in '69 so I figure we're here to stay by now. Virtually all my life I've been involved in selling as a representative for quite a varied type of industries and I've always enjoyed it and the management in the later years and having my own business, and I've been retired now just about 17 years. I'm beginning to like that also and getting used to it.

It's a great time of life, I know certain people retire and they're almost lost for something to do but, to me, I just enjoyed it. Touch wood, I'm still enjoying what I did 40 years ago, probably not quite so agile but still enjoying sailing and hobbies that we do. I'm in the Wooden Boat Association, which I joined just before retirement.

Secret of a happy life

Ron: So certainly retirement hasn't been a problem, I find it great. I've had a good family.

My wife is into golf so 2 days a week she's off playing golf. I think it's also interesting that, as you grow older, you do have individual interests. We get on extremely well still, after 56 years, so I guess that's the secret of a happy life.

Introducing Larry

Larry: I'm Larry Loveday. I was born in Queensland, so I'm a born and bred Queenslander one might say. I'm 85 now, I have a wife who's 2 years older. I began teaching in 1949 at a school in Toowoomba and I worked there for the next 44 and a bit years and I retired in 1993.

We had inherited a property on the coast at Redcliffe, on the beach, and we realised we couldn't maintain two places. So, my wife was very keen to go to the Redcliffe place, where she had spent a lot of time as a girl. So we went there in 1994 and rebuilt what had been a fishing shack, for practical purposes, into a house that was a little more comfortable and we have decided that's where we want to be for as long as we can be.

Joining the Wooden Boat Association

Larry: I joined the Wooden Boat Association shortly after we left Toowoomba. So that would've been about 20 odd years ago.

Keeping busy in retirement

Larry: I have lots of things to keep me busy in my retirement; the maintenance of the boat is one thing. We have a bit of ground so there's grass to mow—I won't call it lawn—and I still keep in touch with the school where I worked for a very long time. I maintain a database about everyone who's ever been there, both students and staff. Until recently I used to do a quarterly journal for the association of the past students; nowadays I sit on the outskirts of it rather more and let other people try and have their fling at it but I still collect information about students who've been there and pass it on to others to write up for the journal.

I enjoy doing all that and I never seem to have enough time to do everything that I aim to do. However, I hope to complete some of these projects before it's time to pass on, as one might say.

Financial challenges and planning for retirement

Ron: Financial challenges since we've been retired were the GFC, that was the global financial scare. We were in England in '09—no, '07 it started—and people were queuing up outside the banks to get their money back and we were a bit concerned.

So we continued to live on our investments that, touch wood, was a reasonable amount that we'd always planned retirement and from the age of about, from certainly from when we were 50, we planned an awful lot from retirement and having adequate income. So it was rather a shock when the GFC did hit Australia and we were on holiday up the Whitsundays and we come home every night and listen to the TV and we were alarmed that the stock market was falling every night and we lost a considerable amount of money over that period which I'm afraid we'll never recover completely, but touch wood that we had sufficient, that really we were able to have a very good lifestyle still.

Failing to plan for the future

Larry: I'm afraid that neither my wife nor I did very much about thinking about plans for the future in our working life. My wife actually stopped work; she was a trained nurse. She actually stopped work after we married and our four sons came along and that was probably just as well; she had her hands full anyway.

So when I retired we had my superannuation, which wasn't a great amount because that particular skill I worked for didn't have superannuation in its schemes until some 20-odd years earlier.

We did have a few investments but not all that much but we've had no real problems so far as living is concerned. Within our limitations, we don't go out every night of the week or anything like that and we've gone past going overseas because we both find that a bit too difficult nowadays, besides the monetary cost of it. So, we have a comfortable life.

Role of the aged carer

Larry: My wife has not been in very good health for some time. Some of my time is taken up as being a carer … I mean, I do the shopping, I escort her wherever it is she needs to go and so on. So some restrictions like that, a new lease of life for her was recently at her 87th birthday her sons gave her a tablet and she now gets up very early in the morning to see what her son, Peter, who lives in Barcelona, has put in his side of the game of Scrabble that they're playing, on the tablet.

Developing computer skills

Larry: I've got reasonable skills on the computer and she is learning very fast, she's way ahead of me as far as the use of the tablet's concerned. I must say though that it has a serious effect on the amount of knitting she's been doing. She has been up till this time been a very enthusiastic and productive knitter. <laughs> For all the grandchildren and their children …

I don't touch her tablet, she doesn't touch my computer. <laughs>

Ron: Yeah, I battled with the computer, with the internet and certain things I'm very happy with. But my wife was a shorthand typist so I don't attempt to do emails as such. I rather take the management lead: I dictate and she does the work and that's a lot quicker because by the time I did an address she would have done the whole thing.

The technological 'time-warp'!

Ron: Over the past 2 months we had to change the television which means a complete new booklet to learn. Then we changed a mobile phone, which once again is not easy. Plus my brother bought me a camera which once again has the menu and everything that opens and closes. I had a laptop for my 80th, so I've been really in a technological kind of time warp that I've almost come to a standstill.

But touch wood, we bought a phone that is extremely good and I will even do SMS messages now … I was able to send photographs to my daughter, so that was a big thrill that I bought a phone that every kind of person of 75 over should have. It is so good and clear and large print … you don't have to put your glasses on to read it.

What we have learned

Larry: I've learnt a lot about, recently, about the genealogical trails, you might say, that you can follow on the computer. They're well-advertised on television, I use a particular one, not the one that's mostly seen on television, I must say and it's very interesting because it provides you with links to families all over the world actually that do have a link with you.

Ron: I know one person who comes sailing and he sets his navigator to find a beach, he then goes out and uses his GPS, so he has a wonderful day out but he doesn't know where he's actually been.

Life doesn't stop when you retire

Ron: There is so much in life which is interesting. I once knew of a manager of ours who retired and drank himself to death within 3 years. That is so tragic, that life doesn't stop just because you retire or you get to be 80. You slow down a bit but really there's still an awful lot to do.

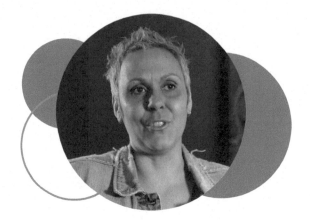

CHAPTER 3

Odette's story

My name is Odette Best. I'm a Wakgun Clan member of the Gorreng Gorreng Nation through my grandmother's bloodline, I'm a Boonthamurra woman through my grandfather's line and my adopted father is a Koomumberri man. So I identify with all three nations.

Looking after ageing Aboriginal people

Like a lot of our Indigenous community members, Aboriginal community members, right across the country, we have got an innate construct to us about looking after our old people.

So, for example, I'm 45 and I am in a middle generation of having two generations below me and two generations above me. So my grandmother is approximately 96 years of age, we're not quite sure, she has three recorded birth dates. She's one of the oldest elders that we actually have in Queensland and essentially is an independent liver.

Historical perspective and repercussions on health

I think, historically, when looking after our ageing Aboriginal population right across the country there is a need for the nursing profession to take better responsibility in understanding Aboriginal health needs for our ageing population.

We've got to remember and realise, as a profession, that our Aboriginal people have actually lived under Acts of administration from 1896, in Queensland, where we were the first state or territory in Australia that ushered in protectionist and segregationist Acts and that was very much an Act in my own family, that my grandmother was removed from country with her mother, my great-grandmother, and removed to a mission outside Rockhampton called Woorabinda. My grandfather, my Boothamurra bloodline, was also removed to that exact same mission.

The missions and reserves across many parts of Australia were operational up until the mid-1970s. So my own family didn't get exempt from the Aboriginal protectionist Acts until 1973.

This particular era, from approximately 1896 until the mid-1970s, left really harsh health impacts on our people so, for example, my grandmother was reared up on a traditional Aboriginal diet that was provided to her by my great-grandmother. But when they got onto the reserves and the missions they were given white flour, white tea, white sugar and bully beef. Now there was real breaking down and severances of traditional diet, lifestyle, spirituality and the whole gamut of cultural constructs for Aboriginal people.

So coming from a very pure and clean diet we were introduced, very harshly, into very processed diets. Now, we have to look at that historical perspective because when you fast-forward it the 40 years or so, the biggest health repercussions that we've actually got in our Aboriginal communities is diabetes and also obesity and also heart disease. And, we now know there is great links between lifestyle—meaning your diet, your exercise, what you do—and the impact of your health.

So nursing, I think as a profession, needs to take a hold of having an historical understanding of some of the health impacts that our older Aboriginal people in our community are actually facing and they have to have an understanding of some of that historical stuff that actually did happen on those Aboriginal people, because they're the Aboriginal people that they're wanting to nurse and look after now in their older life.

Access to health services

So, for example, my own mother had two of her Aboriginal children removed because we were all wards of the state in the 50s and the 60s, 40s and 30s in Queensland. So there's a real reticence for some Aboriginal people to actually access mainstream healthcare services now.

Unfortunately, we don't actually ever look at the service provision of the service, but we look at the people or the community and we do blame them for their non-compliance without having an historical understanding as to why some older Aboriginal people don't access the health services.

So nursing and Aboriginal people, by and large, not all, but by and large, has got a pretty dicey type of history.

Cultural awareness versus cultural sensitivity

I think, importantly, we need to be able to move on from cultural awareness into cultural sensitivity. What cultural awareness actually does for us, is that it allows us the nurse to understand how our healthcare system was set up, why our healthcare system was set up and the treatment that it actually impacted on non-white people. So we start to understand that there are differences between Indigenous people, non-Indigenous people in a cultural awareness type setting.

We can then progress on to becoming culturally sensitive and that's to understand that the differences between Indigenous people and non-Indigenous people are actually really legitimate differences. We can't nurse everybody the same and nor should we try to nurse everybody the same but the profession has really done that here within Australia and it's very problematic for many, many Aboriginal people.

Our old tongues, as we call them in my grandmother's way of speaking, they're called old tongues, they will still not be able to safely go into a hospital because of that historical impact on their health.

Construction of ageing—eldership

The construction of ageing, I believe, between Aboriginal people and non-Aboriginal people in Australia is one of great difference. For many of the Aboriginal communities across Australia eldership is revered and highly regarded so we don't, where we can, separate our elders and our community from the generations that are actually running behind them. So a very few of our Indigenous people actually go into aged care facilities and need to be cared for within their homes, because overwhelmingly we know that a lot of non-Indigenous people actually want to stay in their homes as well and that's the same for Indigenous people but I think what the difference is, is that as our community gets older they reach eldership status and are incredibly highly regarded. They are the knowledge keepers for us, they are the language keepers for us, they're the story keepers for us, they're the law keepers for us.

So the older our Aboriginal population gets, is the more highly regarded they are for their longevity, for their stories and for their lived experiences.

So it's very, very important for, for example, my grandmother, to have the four generations that actually run behind her being very active sources in her life and for her to continue to pass on the knowledge of her lived experience, her language, her law, her country and her boundaries for the generations that come under them. We actually highly revere that knowledge and I don't think that kind of context is quite in the non-Indigenous community as it is in the Aboriginal community.

So you'll find that our elders within our communities are usually incredibly supported by their own direct descendancy but also the broader community. So, for example, in a number of our communities right across Queensland we have very active and up-and-running elders groups. I'll be honest, they are treated like royalty, and it's a real pride for our communities to be able to have our elders, as few as we've actually got, to be there and to pass on their knowledge.

Becoming recognised as an elder

How do you become recognised as an elder? That's through each individual community that they particularly live in, for example, so it's not that you hit the age of 55 and you automatically become an elder. Traditionally, elders were known within their communities for their knowledge, their language, their law, their customs, their culture and that type of stuff. So for us in our communities it's not a number that you hit, where you hit eldership status, you have to be recognised within your own community for those things I've just rattled off to reach eldership status.

We don't have a golden number in our community context that says 'you're an elder now'. So with the life differential of Indigenous and non-Indigenous people in the country, it's a rarity to have Indigenous people, Aboriginal people who are well into their 70s, 80s and 90s and it's more uncommon than it is common. So they are highly regarded within our communities, but it's not a digit for us, it's not a number that makes you an elder. It's your knowledge!

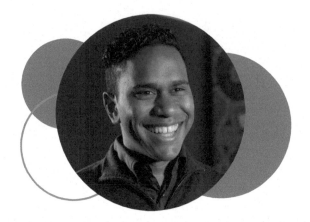

CHAPTER 3

Ali's story

My name's Ali Drummond. I'm a Torres Strait Islander. It means that I'm from the Torres Straits, so that's in Northern Queensland so a group of islands between Queensland and Papua New Guinea. I'm also a registered nurse.

Caring for my grandparents at home

During my time growing up in the Torres, I also had obligations as a young person, growing in a house with my grandparents and caring for them as well in home. So caring for older people in my family has not always been in an established institute, it's been outside of aged care homes as well. So, it's been a regular or a normal duty.

Roles and responsibilities in the Torres Strait Islander community

Like many roles within the Torres Strait Islander community, the roles and responsibilities around supporting our elders or older people as they age and experience health conditions that are more common in our older people. So there's roles and responsibilities around that, and I think there's always been that sense of, say obligation—obligation seems like a strong word or there's a sense of someone not wanting to do it. But, I think within the Torres Strait Islander community there's a loving obligation so it is our role just like it's the role of the elders to contribute to community.

Health services and the home

I grew up in my maternal grandmother's house and her mother—so, my great-grandmother—was still alive when I was growing up. So I still recall fond memories of my great-grandmother and how she was cared for by my mum and my aunties. So was my grandmother when she was going through the end stage of her life. There was very little, I guess, contact, that I can remember, with the health service for my great-grandmother and maybe because of the experience of her, her own experience as well as my grandmother's experience growing up in the Torres under multiple government policies. So, for them, there was still that distrust that they had with the health service. My great-grandmother spent a lot of time at home, especially at the end stage of her life. So I remember those experiences.

I've also lost my grandfather from my mum's side, so my maternal grandfather, and the end stage of his life he spent at home as well and my mother played a huge role in caring for him at home. My mum's a health worker and she's also worked as an AIN at the local hospital so she knew the basic nursing care, but outside of that, it was more about the social and the cultural factors, I think, so it was an opportunity for the family to come together for an environment that wasn't an institution like a hospital or an aged home where they could share this very significant time with my grandfather.

Caring for my grandfather

So the experience I've had with my grandfather from my dad's side, so my paternal grandfather, he turned 96 this year and it's only been the last 5 years where he's been more of a home body, not by choice though. Most of his life, since he retired in the late 60s, he's been a fisherman. So he went fishing every day except Sundays. Sunday was church day so we would go to church with him. But every other day we'd go fishing; well, if we could, if we didn't have school, we'd go fishing with him. So, he's been pretty independent most of his life.

So during that period of going from his 60s through to his 90s, he would, every now and then, have health issues. His gout, I think, was his biggest enemy, because he just loves to eat and he's just so used to eating so many different cuisines because, well, up in the Torres we have such a mixture of culture and so Malaysian food, Japanese food: he is no stranger to eating or even cooking those kinds of cuisines. So they were often terrible for his gout, so he'd never find out until the next day so sometimes he'd get really bad and he'd just refuse to go into hospital for care.

I remember a lot of times actually caring for him, you know, assisting him to the toilet, helping him shower, even bed bathing him at home so even before even considering a career in nursing these were things that we did. I guess for me at the time it just didn't seem unnatural, it was something that I was asked to do by my parents and then my grandfather needed to have happen and because he has a role in teaching me how to fish and telling me about his experiences and what he's learnt in life and all, the values he's learnt. It was an opportunity again, I guess, to learn more about his life but also to do something that he actually needed.

68

Working as an AIN

These experiences that I've had with my grandparents were valuable when I went into aged care, working as an AIN. For me the important thing wasn't the clinical stuff that needed to get done, for me the important thing was actually listening to the stories, spending time with all the people. I know with some of the elders that they had family members that hadn't visited in a month or 2 months so you get that sense of loneliness that they felt. So just having someone listen about something as simple as how their day went and how much they didn't like their dinner meant a lot for them. So, it wasn't just about getting them showered and ready for breakfast: those are the sorts of things that can happen during the course of the day.

It was about making sure that they were keen, mentally and psychologically as well, that they were getting their needs met there. I guess, culturally, I was lucky, or maybe I like to think my grandparents felt lucky that they spent more time at home with family and unfortunately for some of the older people that I was caring for they had to move off their islands to move to TI, to be cared for, for many reasons.

But there was a sense of disconnection from country or from community from not being able to see the view of the beach that they had when they were back at home, not having to taste, you know, the local foods like sardines, fish, turtle, turtle egg that you could just get because someone next door would've gone out and got you some. You don't have that in an institution like that, so for me, I really, really felt for the oldies that I looked after and it was just, how they just talked so fondly about their community. That really touched me and, I guess, helped me see the other side of nursing which is about the people and their experiences.

Chronic disease in the community

We all know that Aboriginal and Torres Strait Islander people suffer a whole lot of chronic disease and do experience premature deaths in compared to non-Indigenous Australians. So for Torres Strait Islander experience, we have a lot of our men and women that are around 30 or 40 that are experiencing these chronic diseases; so, much earlier than their non-Indigenous counterparts.

My dad, for example, he has a number of health problems but he's really reluctant to go see anyone about it. A lot of his generation of friends and family members and my mum, as well, have a number of health problems that they're battling with. So for Torres Strait Islanders, I think, in regards to ageing and health deterioration, that happens a whole lot earlier, I think, for Torres Strait Islanders or in my family at least. So we do experience a lot of chronic diseases earlier.

From a cultural or a social perspective, I guess more from the social perspective unfortunately it has become seen as the norm. So for a lot of Torres Strait Islander people around that age, unfortunately, that's become accepted as the norm. So, someone gets gout, like I said before, high blood pressure, ya know, it's not a big issue, unfortunately. I think that's a scary thing, not only for my dad, my mum, their generation but also for the younger people coming through and I guess being exposed to these ideals that it is normal to be overweight or greater than that or to engage in risk-taking behaviours that lead to early onset of these chronic diseases.

Barriers to optimal healthcare

One of the biggest barriers in regards to optimal healthcare for the ageing, especially for Torres Strait Islander people that are ageing, I think, lies in the history. Specifically in the Torres, we've had … I've mentioned before quite a long history of imposing policies and I think it's important for anyone working within the sector to appreciate that. A lot of our older people and even those a bit younger than the older people have experienced at least some time under these policies, so for them they didn't have the opportunities that they do now. I mentioned how my great-grandmother and my grandmother have this distrust—my grandmother today still has this distrust—that creates this huge barrier for her accessing healthcare. She's at home at the moment, my grandmother, she's living at home with one of my cousins, early onset dementia, she has a number of chronic diseases. She refuses, no matter how hard the local health service tries—they even visit her home—she refuses to even engage with them because she's had that ingrained in her since she was little.

I think one of the biggest issues is that, for someone who is currently working in the sector or planning to work in the sector and will be looking after a Torres Strait Islander, and possibly Aboriginal people as well, it's important to remember that our older people lived through these experiences, these policies.

So I guess that's the first stage, for institutions and health workers—whether they are Indigenous, non-Indigenous—to actually think about what these other people have experienced.

Cultural and social infrastructure

So the second thing is, is optimising the cultural mechanisms or the social infrastructure that's in place in the Torres Strait Islander communities already. So not every Torres Strait Islander community will still practise looking after their old people at home but a lot will. So it's speaking with the family that you're engaged with around, you know, what kind of support have you or do you intend to provide for the older person that's going to be in your care. So whether it's in your acute setting, so if an older lady or gentleman's coming in for a fractured mouth they'll still need that support as well as in an aged care setting.

So it's talking to the family about how can nursing care and nursing interventions be complemented by what's already existing in the family and not shutting them out and seeing them as someone that comes during visiting hours, because these are the people that provide that really important cultural connection still.

Torres Strait Islander history and culture

I'm not sure how familiar people are with Torres Strait Islander history but we have had a number of visitors, we've had religion come in and embed itself quite strongly in our culture so people say that we've been colonised by religion but we've also had the governments.

Today we have this younger generation that have had more privileges and have been more accepted in Australian community than any generation of Torres Strait Islander community.

Now this is an important thing to remember … so for the older people that you're actually caring for they've never had these, or they've had limited experiences that the younger generation have, definitely have had today. They've been excluded from society so they've not had the educational opportunities, not had the employment opportunities that a lot of Australians have today. So these things have informed their life.

So now we're here and we have all these opportunities and a lot of things have been recognised and there has been an apology but these older people still have experiences.

You can't assume someone's a Torres Strait Islander because they look Torres Strait Islander because there's no particular look in the last 200 history. We haven't just been visited by England; we've been visited by Malaysian, Japanese and people from the South Pacific, PNG. People from PNG and Aboriginal people we've always been engaged in. There's not one look Torres Strait Islander people, there's not one culture. It's quite a smorgasbord so for health professionals looking after older people it's good to get to know the person you're looking after, so get to know their background. Just don't assume that just because they're a Torres Strait Islander they eat and hunt turtle and dugong or all this other stuff that … these are assumptions that I've come across introducing myself as a Torres Strait Islander. Get to know them.

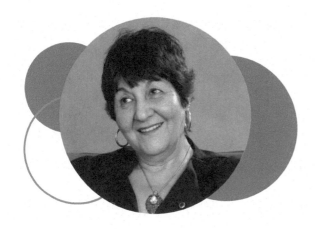

CHAPTER 4

Mercedes' story

I'm Mercedes Sepulveda. I've been in Australia for 25 years and I'm a social scientist from a Chilean background.

I've been working in the multicultural area for about … 20 years.

Ageing versus ageism

If we look at culture in Australia but in terms of ageing, I could say we need to consider and look at first, ageism, which is different to ageing. What I have noticed in this country, but I think it's around the world, is that ageism is impacting on older people because of the systematic stereotyping and discrimination towards old people. So there is a culture of ageism, and it's important to notice that ageing is a natural process of getting older, but ageism sometimes is impacting on how people could age happily and healthily.

Ageism for me is a systemic stereotyping and discrimination towards older people and ageing is just a natural process of getting older. And it's just how your body is changing and how your abilities are changing, but it's just a natural process. Because in ageing, since you were born you are already ageing, so it's just a process.

Challenges of ageing

Ageing in a different culture involves a lot of challenges and I don't think Australia is actually addressing those challenges. There are a lot of issues that haven't been taken into consideration, like cultural differences, working with diversity, language issues, communication and discrimination and isolation.

Australia is a multicultural society

Australia needs to recognise and act upon that Australia is a multicultural society, because 25% of the population—from the current census—identified that 25% of the population was born overseas. And also the last census identified that there are people … from 200 different countries and 200 different languages. So you can't, in a multicultural society, have just one set of services or with a mentality of 'one size fits all', because of the diversity that exists.

We need to look at diversity

We need to look at the diversity of how people came to Australia, so there are people who came at a younger age, so they could adapt, maybe, or settle quicker and also learn the language. There are other people who arrive in Australia and there are older people who arrive in Australia, so how they settle and how they manage this ageing process is totally different. On the other hand, we need to look at that there were people who came as migrants, there were people who came as refugees onshore and offshore. So when I'm saying onshore, I'm talking about asylum seekers, but also I'm talking about refugees offshore; that means that they were already recognised overseas to come to Australia as a refugee.

So all of these impact on how people settle and their experience in ageing, because some people manage the language, some people have difficulties in learning the language—at a mature age it's more difficult—and there are some people who just survive with the language or just manage, but during the whole process of time, and it's just a survival level.

Accessing services

Accessing services is one of the biggest issues and because services and staff are not equipped for trying to work with diversity. So language is one of the biggest barriers and not many services use interpreters and also not many people are aware of the services available to them because it hasn't been in their native language or if there is, say, translated information, we are assuming that everybody is literate in English or in another language.

So, yes, that is the biggest issue, community services are not using as they should interpreters, and also other ways of disseminating information to people, on the one side. And on the other side is that, as I said, people's attitudes. I'm talking about the three levels of services: government, non-government and community services, where still people haven't addressed the issue of working with diversity, so there is a lot of stereotyping, discrimination and expecting assimilation rather than working with diversity.

Cultural sensitivity

Say, for example, this was a family from the horn of Africa, just an example of how the hospital, for example, wasn't responding in a culturally sensitive way and with competence. It was child number seven, I think, of that family that was coming to this world and so the mother was suggested to go to the hospital for a check-up and then in that check-up the nurse I imagine was, I'm not 100% sure who actually told the person the sex of the baby, and that was detrimental because in that culture you can't know. And it was detrimental to the extent that they needed counselling support and, again, another barrier there because counselling wasn't something that they practised either. So as a worker, I have to start looking at how and what will be the best way to support this family with this process. So I'm telling you that because I experienced that and I was involved in that case.

The multicultural framework and self-awareness

'Culture' is very hard to define as well, because there are more than 120 definitions of 'culture'. However, if professionals and staff are able to practise what is called multicultural practice framework, they will be able to work with everybody, they wouldn't be assuming or judging, they would be checking, asking, valuing the experience of people and the culture of other people.

It's impossible that we can know about every culture but we can acquire—and this is why cultural competency is very important—to know how to work with and how to involve people from other cultures in the process.

The basis of the multicultural framework is that the individual or the worker or the practitioner, if I can put it in that way, actually needs to be aware of themselves; self-awareness is critical. They need to understand their own cultural beliefs and values and, if they understand themselves, they will be able to understand others.

People need to do self-awareness and then, if they do the self-awareness training, they can go into understanding the multicultural practice framework. Once they understand that framework, they will be able to understand working with diversity, but working with diversity not just practitioners and clients, this is in the whole society, all right, and in the bigger context. So when they do that and they experience working with people, they could work with everybody. So that's what is expected when you practise that framework.

Aged care reform and multicultural strategies

If this aged care reform is going to make a difference, and I imagine this is what it's there for, and now that they include the culturally and linguistically diverse multicultural strategy, it is possible that, because it's included, there is an expectation that the issues that culturally and linguistically diverse background people are facing can be addressed.

Training is one of the very important components in this reform and it is also suggested in the strategy how to do it.

So how I see this happening is if, you know, whoever is implementing it needs to be monitored. It needs to be monitored how service providers are meeting needs based on this strategy, otherwise it could be going around and around. And also resources need to be put towards this in order to address that, because the use of interpreters has been always an issue for services, because they haven't been funded to do so and, while my issue is, well, if this reform is for everybody, all of these components need to be included in there, otherwise, as I said, it's going to be marginalising again this group which is already considered as a special group.

So for how long, my question is, is this going to be considered a special group if they are not doing a real intervention in order to address this? So I'm expecting, and I'm very hopeful, that by having this strategy included into the reform, I think there is more potential. And I would like also an entity like the Federation of Community Councils of Australia to actually monitor how this strategy is being implemented into the reform and how it is implemented also in the funding bodies' agreements. I think that could be a way of making a difference.

Services are for everybody

My vision is not to segregate the community, it's just to be part of the whole community and so every service is actually addressing all the needs, regardless of what age you are, if you are from a particular background or because you speak another language at home. So that's what I envisage to see: is that the services are for everybody and no segregating and putting as a special group, or having special programs to address multicultural issues when it should be included in the whole spectrum of services, I would say.

CHAPTER 4

Rafael's story

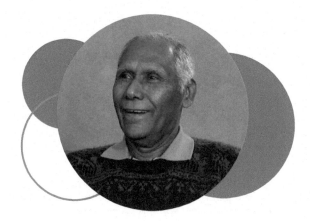

My name is Rafael. I was born in El Salvador. I've been living in Australia for 28 years with my family; it's my wife and three children. I am a pensioner now, but I've been working, yeah, up to last year, working as an accountant.

I'm 71, yeah.

Coming to Australia

We were living in Costa Rica, a neighbouring country of El Salvador in Central America, and we knew about the special program called Special Humanitarian Program for refugees living outside the country, let's say, in Costa Rica, and we applied to come to Australia. And we arrived in Melbourne in 1984 and, after 1 year living in Melbourne, we decided to move to Brisbane, and we have been living in Brisbane for the last 27 years.

We had already the experience of being 12 years in Costa Rica, which the situation was more difficult, then coming to Australia was easy from the economic perspective, the security, because we came as permanent residents, which means that we had all the rights, or most of the rights, of an Australian citizen. And that made life easier. At the time, there was migrant hostels in which all migrants were in, and that facilitated our settling-in process, because there were all kinds of services in those migrant hostels.

So we spent 7 months in the migrant hostel in Melbourne … learning another language, knowing about the new culture, from that perspective, yes, of course, we confronted a lot of difficulties that we had to overcome, especially the language barrier.

Learning the English language

At the migrant hostel, the English classes were given very … I mean, in the same compound, so we just had to go from our flat into the English classes, which were very, very close, and that facilitated us to be together and to learn, to start learning the language.

There were different levels, so we had to pass a test first to see which level, which is, you know, intermediate and advanced and beginners. But I never imagined how difficult it is to learn a second language when you are … I was 42 when I came to Australia, as you know, the older you are, the more difficult it is to learn anything, not only languages, but to learn anything.

I could see my friends, I used to have a lot of friends from El Salvador coming together. Even the plane in which we came, it was full of El Salvadorans, there were about more than 50 of us in the same plane, and we became friends in the migrant hostel. And we used to talk about that, the different levels of education, the different levels of travelling and all that makes a lot of difference. And age is, you know … I saw people of 50 years old and they couldn't … they couldn't learn the language, they just learnt some words, but they couldn't. And also the level of education makes a difference.

Language barriers and jobs

I saw many professionals that couldn't overcome the language problem and they couldn't go into work into their profession, yeah, and that is very frustrating. I suppose, because I was able, after two and a half years, to work in my profession, yes, and that is very important, very rewarding for one person to know that, 'Yes, I am working in my profession'; that is something that helped me so much, not only financially but also in the aspect of the self-esteem is lifted by having a job in your profession.

Raising children and grandchildren

As a grandfather within my family, we more or less support our children in raising their children. And that's very good for a retired person like me, because I can see my grandchildren being, you know, raised in a different way, of course.

In our time, it was different: we were punished physically and all that, but now you can't do that, and things like that, you know, you have to understand, you have to accept and be intelligent enough to understand that time passes and that we can't stick in the past, we can't live in the past, we have to learn new things. And that learning process has a lot to see with what I was talking to you about being … working in your profession, finding a job, being within your community and go within the mainstream community and be accepted and all that.

Settling in and frustrations

I have seen people, very successful people who speak the language very quickly, and people who have been frustrated because they can't do it. I mean, they are stuck there, for any reason, and those people, they live a bad life. Sometimes they even have gone back thinking that they are living a very bad life here emotionally. And what happened is that they come back again and back, and they are back and forth, and their life is almost wrecked by not being able to settle in properly, you know, not only economically, but mainly emotionally, this is the main problem. Because in here, I remember we had a Housing Commission house, which is decent, a very decent house, in which we were feeling very well.

So it is not about the living conditions, the physical living conditions, but it's more about the emotional part of how you feel in the society. That's really, really essential to feel that you are part, to feel that your self-esteem is really raised. Because the first thing that the migrant loses is self-esteem because we start to think, 'Am I able to do this? Is my experience going to be good enough in this new environment? In my profession, am I going to perform very well if I got a job?', and that is something that affects many people. Once you overcome that problem, then you are okay.

And I have seen cases, even of suicide: there has been at least one case in my community of a professional committing suicide because he couldn't stand it, and he couldn't go back because his family was here.

Accessing social services

If I compare the social services in my country to the ones in Australia, I'll say there is no comparison. I mean, here you've got access to a lot of services. However, once you are here, you have to have information, you have to know that the services are there and to do that you need to go to the street, to talk to people, to visit places, not be isolated in your house, which is very common in migrants. They usually feel safe within their houses.

There was a situation in which I became more a community worker rather than an accountant, yes, and people used to call me, 'Rafael, do you know where I can find this?' and I knew usually; and even, I tell you, some people who were born here. I was working for a community legal service for 11 years and when I talked to mainstream people about 'Do you know about what community legal services are in Brisbane?' and they don't know, and I got all the lists of the community legal services and I used to give the addresses, telephone numbers to my friends who to go to if you have a problem. 'Did you have a car accident? Okay, go to this legal service, they're going to help you.' So I had the information because I knew that information, knowledge, is power. And then that empowers you to live in a new society.

That made it, for me, easier but at the same time I was aware how so many people didn't know how to access those services. It is a problem from the service providers; they have to find another way, how to pass the information to the people in need.

Children as interpreters

If they speak the language, it is easier, but if they don't then it's really difficult because they have to stay within their community; they are unable to go by themselves to other places, they need a person to accompany them, usually their children. I remember in Melbourne, because the children pick up the language so easily, and so the parents used to bring their children to the doctor, to the hospital, to everywhere as interpreters.

And the children, of course, are not trained to be interpreters, and so the parents were dependent on their children. And that is a very bad relationship; the children miss the authority: 'Who's got the power here? I've got the power because I speak English, you know, so my parent is not as clever as I thought' and things like that. So for older people coming here and not speaking the language, it's frustrating, it's a way of being isolated and not developing their personality properly.

New process of learning

Coming from a society like ours in which men are the ones with the power, the macho society, even when personally I haven't been that sort of macho, however, it is impossible not to have that influence. And, for instance, to do housework duties, I didn't do anything back in El Salvador, not even the first years here.

Then I have learnt to do house duties like cooking, like washing, like cleaning the house. My wife is working, it will be unfair for me just to stay home and her come in to do the food. And so that is a new process of learning which I value and I appreciate so much because it has given me the opportunity to be fair within my own home, within my own family.

Accepting the challenge of getting older

Learning, accepting new challenges, accepting the challenge of getting older; the process of getting older is the most difficult thing that you can imagine, because then you can see the end of your life as a reality, not as when you are 20 that you think you will be eternal. But now, after 70, you say, 'God, usually people live to 80' so if my average will be 80, say, it's only 10 years, and what sort of life, what quality of life? Because it is not only life, you can be living with oxygen, and that's not life. I mean, quality of life: going out, we still go out with my wife for dancing parties and, of course, we are not going to discos, but we go out to family reunions, and I still have my glass of wine whenever I want. And so we try to enjoy life within all the problems that we can have.

And the other thing is trying to help, trying to assist my community; that has given me that power. Every time I am able to do something for other families, I am talking about advice, accompanying them, to be with them, quality of my time, not the time that I don't use, but quality of time to be with them. And knowing that those words were good for them, that again gives me, you know, the reason to continue the same way, the 'same way' meaning learning, changing, every day changing … changing the old patterns to improve ourselves. If we stay still then there is no progress.

It is the same with the societies. The societies go further and further forward, so the person has to be the same, we have to think, we have to open our minds and serve other people; for my wife and myself, that is a must.

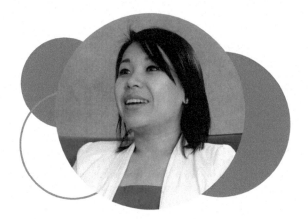

CHAPTER 5

Cindy's story

I'm Dr Cindy Jones. I'm a research fellow doing research in the area of dementia, and my area of dementia research focuses on relationship, sexuality in residential aged care.

Sexuality as a multidimensional construct

Often if you ask somebody what sexuality is, they will tell you, 'Oh, it's about sexual orientation'. But in fact the term 'sexuality' is actually a much broader concept. It actually is a multidimensional construct, because it actually involves things like gender identity and role, and it also includes a person's need for love, affection, companionship, relationship, as well as a need for intimacy. Young people often have this prevailing ageist view that older people and sexuality doesn't go hand-in-hand, and they like to think that older people can't have sex, aren't interested in sex, or is a sexual human being, and we know that that is not true. And this view is so prevailing that often older people can't actually express their sexual needs or desire.

Challenges and barriers to sexual expression

The challenges or the barriers for older people expressing themselves sexually in both residential and community area would be things like the lack of an able partner, so the lack of a partner that can express sexually, or express themselves sexually, and it could also be to … it could also be due to medication that they might be taking that can actually prevent them to be performing sexual activities.

Issue of privacy

With aged care facility there's the issue of privacy, because you are in a residential care environment, the issue of privacy where nurses often walk into rooms without knocking can be a real concern when they are wanting to engage in sexual activities, whereas in your home environment in your community, you can do it in the privacy of your own home, without someone walking in through the door and intruding on you.

Residential versus community environment

In residential aged care facility as well, the difference is that family and care staff often have a very paternalistic view and role, that because you're in an aged care facility we have to look after you, we have to be concerned about your benefit, and the risk involved if you wish to express yourself sexually. Whereas in a community environment, that often doesn't happen because there is no one to curtail you as to what you are doing in your own home.

Information on sexual expression

As far as I'm aware, there hasn't been any specific resources, pamphlet or information sheet that is available for older people regarding sexual expression. And there was a study that was conducted a few years ago with a questionnaire that was sent out to all residential aged care facilities, as well as community aged care services, to ask them if they were doing anything to actually promote, or give information about, sexuality and older people, specifically about sexual expression for older people. And the outcome of that study was that there wasn't many response to that questionnaire. And it suggests two things. The first thing is number one that there is nothing out there whatsoever; number two, this is a topic of area which is so sensitive that aged care service provider, whether it's community or residential aged care, it's not something they want to talk about very much.

Older people's ability to discuss sexual preferences

What we know based on talking with older people is that older people often wish to discuss their sexual needs and desire with a healthcare professional, as to how to approach healthcare professionals to raise their concern with them, because they feel … they are concerned about the ageist view that can actually apply for health professional, they are worried that health professional might think that they are different, or they might see them as being the dirty old person, or dirty old man, or the dirty old woman, wanting to talk about sexual needs and concerns. So that inhibits them from raising their concern with health professional, despite them wishing and wanting the opportunity to talk to healthcare professionals about it.

And on the other side, for healthcare professional, even though for those that do recognise that older people do have sexual needs and desire, and wish to talk about their concern, they often feel uncertain and not trying in actually discussing about sexual needs and concerns with older people. So as a result of it, they don't actually talk about it as part of their normal care assessment, or normal care for older people when it comes to sexuality.

LGBTI community and inclusivity

The LGBTI community is now calling for inclusive aged care service, that irregardless of gender orientation or gender identities or roles, that the care provision will be the same for every older person that is admitted to aged care, or is receiving community care. Unfortunately at this stage, when you talk to care staff the issue of caring for someone of the same ... or the issue of caring for someone from the LGBTI community is of real concern, because they might say, oh yes, they are okay with it, but when time comes to crunch for them to be caring for someone from the LGBTI community, often what we find is that care staff are quite uncomfortable due to a lack of knowledge, due to a lack of understanding, and due to a lack of training of how to respond to the needs for members of the LGBTI community.

So what we are hoping to see is that there will be change through education and training, that care staff will be ... care staff or health professional will have a better understanding of the needs of older people in terms of sexual expression, irregardless whether they are heterosexual, or they belong from the LGBTI community, and they will be all treated with respect, their sexual orientation, sexual preferences, sexual expression will be treated with respect and dignity, and they will be given the space, the room to express themselves however they wish to, as long as it does not actually impede on the space or the rights of other people in the share community.

Challenges for care staff

We have care staff that come from a multicultural and ethnic background that is really challenging for them to accept residents or older people that is from the LGBTI community, because there is for them, for their own culture, or from their own ethnic background ... LGBTI is not well or commonly accepted to be the norm.

Unfortunately, times are changing. At the moment in aged care we have older people that are quite conservative in nature. However, we have the '60s and the '70s sexual revolution, and those are the group that are fast ageing, and those are the next group of ageing population that we're going to have, and they are the one that will be requiring care. They are going to be admitted to an aged care facility, or receiving community care, and they will not be appreciative of care staff or health professional telling them how they can express themselves sexually, what is considered the norm, or what is considered acceptable within a care environment, and they definitely will not be putting up with their family members telling them what they can or can't do.

As I say to others, just imagine your aged care facility having people like Mick Jagger, people like Elton John coming in aged care, receiving care. Are you going to be telling them what they can or can't do? Whether what they can or can't express themselves in terms of sexual needs, and desire, and preferences? So think about that. And at the end of the day, it will focus on person-centred care, we need to address the needs of our clients, how we can better support them in sexual expression so that they it actually gives rise, or enhances their overall wellbeing and quality of life.

Safe, acceptable environments

It will be a place where we're going to have a group of older people that can have different sexual orientation, that it will be an environment where they feel safe, they will feel accepted, for old ... it will be for older people to feel safe and accepted, and that they are respected, whichever their sexual orientation may be, or however their sexual orientation may be. And it's also about a workplace that is actually proactive in supporting older people in their sexual expression, rather than reactive.

Guidelines and policies

And it is also about a workplace having clear guidelines and policy as to how they can support older people in their sexual expression. And what you will find right now is a lot of organisation, or aged care organisation, do not have any policy or guidelines for staff in terms of how they should respond, or even assess older people that have sexual ... that is actually expressing themselves sexually.

Cognitive capacity to consent

Now the other thing that we need to consider is the issue of dementia. A lot of older people who are admitted to aged care facility, a large proportion of them do have dementia. Now if you join the issue of dementia plus sexual expression, it adds on another layer of complexity, because this time now is not just about expressing themselves sexually, it's about their cognitive capacity to consent to a new relationship, to consent to a new sexual relationship. And because we often feel, or we often view older people who have dementia to be vulnerable, that needs to be looked after, we are often worried that if they enter into a new relationship, especially if it's sexual, is the person with dementia able to give consent, or are they coerced, or are they actually duped into a sexual relationship?

An example

Let me give you an example. There was this incident of this older lady that formed a sexual relationship with this older gentleman. Now she appears to give signs of consent, and verbal and physical body language to suggest that she's quite happy to go along with the gentleman into his room, and engage in sexual activity, and staff can see that from her behaviour. However, the concern that staff have for her because she has dementia was that every time after a sexual encounter with the older person, or with the gentleman in question, when she comes out from it, she often seems to look distressed, and emotionally disturbed, and hurt, and despair. And upon investigation what staff members found was that every time after a sexual episode or a sexual encounter she has with the gentleman, the gentleman will simply leave her, and ask her to leave his room.

So whilst the staff recognise that she has given consent to give—to actually have that sexual encounter with the gentleman—but what the staff actually recognise is signs of ill-being after the sexual encounter for the person, for the lady with dementia, because she doesn't understand that the gentleman is using her simply as a sexual partner, with no intention to form any further intimate relationship, which is obviously what she's craving.

So while she might have given all the signs of verbal consent to this sexual relationship, but she doesn't seem to recognise the consequences, or the emotional despair she is actually experiencing, because the next time it happens, she forgets about how she felt after having the sexual encounter. So as a result the staff have to intervene and put a stop to the continuation of this sexual relationship, because it's not to the benefit of the lady due to the size of ill-being that she displays after the sexual encounter.

Current research into the need for intimacy and sexual expression

We know from the statistics as well is that from a study in the US that looked at sexual activities, sexual behaviour and sexual problem of the adult population, what it was found was that for older adults between the age of 65 to 74, over 50% indicated that they are still engaging in sexual activity, and this result is similar to a study in Australia that was done in over … in nearly 2000 men who is over the age of 65. And what they found as well was that close to or up to 50% of men that is between the age of 75 to 95 have indicated that sex continued to be a somewhat important topic in their life, and that they continued to have this desire and needs.

But unfortunately there has been a real lack of study in the area of sexual behaviour for the adult, or for the older female population. But definitely all the evidence out there seems to suggest that sexual expression does not end when they reach a certain age; in fact, it continues. And what we also know is that while sexual activity do decline with age, we recognise that it does decline with age; however, the need for intimacy, the need for affection, companionship, the need to have a loving, intimate relationship with another human being remains, and it continues to exist, doesn't matter what age you are.

Understanding sexual orientation, needs and desires

Keep an open mind. Understand, respect that everyone's sexual orientation, everybody's sexual needs and desire are different, that we are all different, individual beings, and that it doesn't matter what age we are, we're all human beings, we do have sexual needs and desire. And I would ask them to put themselves in a role where they're in their 60s and 70s, and they at that point in time imagine them continuing wanting to have that desire, or having the need for sexual expression, and someone coming in and telling them what they can or can't do, or someone actually ridiculing them, or laughing, or making some negative remarks about their behaviour, how would that feel? Because then that will keep … that will actually make them understand exactly what they're doing to older people who are wishing to express themselves sexually right now, because then that will make them think about how they are responding to older people expressing themselves sexually. And we recognise that every one of us, every individual, do have views and opinion about how someone should behave, but we shouldn't form a judgement, and we shouldn't let that affect the quality of care provision that we provide to our residents, the quality of care provision we provide to older people that is dependent on us for their care provision.

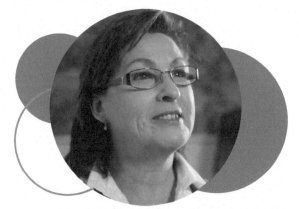

CHAPTER 6

Theresa's story

My name's Theresa, and I'm a nurse and I work full-time. I'm also a carer. I'm a carer of my elderly mother, who's got a lot of co-morbidities, meaning that she has many illnesses, and needs lots of support, and she lives with me. I also have a young adult boy at home. When I say young, he's 20, and he has a learning disability so he needs lots of support and direction in life. I also have a married daughter, and a beautiful little granddaughter.

When I think about the sorts of things I need to do for my son, it's not just supporting him—he's at university—and directing him, and keeping him on task. But it's also making sure he's eating, making sure that he's got transport to where he needs to go. So he is quite dependent on me. Then my mother is also very dependent on me, emotionally.

I would be at work full-time and she would ring me, and I'd be in the middle of a meeting and she'd go, 'I'm having difficulty breathing'. And I would be there, like, trying to do my job, at the same time as then thinking, 'Well, Mum, I'll ring you back in a minute, take some deep breaths, you know, get onto your Ventolin, I'll be with you soon'.

Sometimes in my career I've said to my husband, 'Maybe I need to give up work, and just stay home and support her' and he and my mother both said, 'No, that's not fair, we wouldn't expect that of you'.

I need to get off this roundabout

So when I think about the emotional support I have to give to my mother, I have to give to my son, then to my daughter, and then to my mother, sometimes I would think, 'I need to get off this roundabout, I can't keep going like this' because it would be constant. I would finish work, go home and then I would need to actually debrief with my mother what sort of day she's had. She'd want to talk to me, and if I didn't feel like talking she'd go, 'Oh, you never to talk to me. I'm always at home all by myself all day and then you don't talk to me'. Then my husband would want me to talk to him as well. And we have an upstairs/downstairs situation, so my mother is upstairs, my husband is downstairs, and Mum would like me to speak to her and my husband would like to speak to me. And so that sometimes my husband would say, 'You've just got home and you spend an hour with your Mother, you haven't even come in and spoken to me'. So again, I'm torn with my emotions, of trying to support everyone and be what they all want me to actually be. And I think that that's where you actually find it really difficult. My daughter's fabulous, she really is good. But again, whenever she asks me to support her, or to look after the baby, I would look after the baby. So sometimes I would have the baby and my mother, and I'd still have to drop Jacob off somewhere or something like that too. So again, it's full-on, and it is quite emotional.

Different roles

When I think about all the different roles that I've actually got to do, I think that that was the best way for me to actually deal with all those different roles was to actually split them up, and think of who I'm trying to be at this particular time. There were times I didn't do it very well. There were times when perhaps there were fights in the house because I was tired, and I was sick of being everything to everyone else. And they wouldn't understand that: they'd just think that I was being grumpy, and that I was going through menopause, and so that's the sort of thing it is. And I knew what it was; it's just emotionally draining trying to be something to everyone. But then I would stop and take a big deep breath and say, 'It is what it is. I love them all, I wouldn't have it any other way. They're my family, so you do what you've gotta do'.

Debriefing

I debrief with colleagues. And I think being able to come to work and just talk about the stresses that I've got at home, when you had a break, gave you that relief. And then you could do your work at work, and be that person you are at work, and go home feeling a little bit refreshed. So although being everything and working full-time, it's not easy, I think that sort of support keeps you going there as well. So, again, understanding those roles, I knew that my work was who I was, so I was able to be Theresa, rather than Pat's daughter, Jacob's mum, George's wife.

But because my mother is still cognitively intact and an intelligent person, she was still mothering me. So even though I was supporting her and being the carer, she was still, in some ways, still being my mother and letting me debrief with her about 'Oh, Jacob's done this, or at work this happened' and she would try and help me resolve it. So I think that was good. If she had've been just dependent on me and not still my mother and not play that role sometimes, I think that would have affected it. But the fact is that she still tried to be that supportive mother at times. But then there would be other times where I'd come home and I'd be a bit down, and she'd ask me what was going on, and she'd listen to me. So I think that that's really important that she was still being that role, and being that person to me.

It is what it is

I know someone said to me once when my mother was constantly staying with me, you know, 'What's gonna happen when she needs more care?' You know, 'What are you going to do? You need to be your own thing'. And I'm going, 'But she's my mother! I'm doing it because she is my mother, that's it!' And I don't mean it was my role, I just knew that this is who I am, this is what I am. She's done so much for me in my life, why would you not support her? It is what it is, and I don't resent it at all. I just think okay, I look back and I think, 'Wow, that was pretty emotional, it was pretty stressful. But I did it, and I learnt more about myself'. And I think that's what life's about. You learn from other people that you care for, about the sort of person you are. It makes you who you are. And I think that that's probably the most significant part about being in the sandwich years, is that if you actually look at it and reflect, and then think, 'Well, what sort of character am I and how am I growing from this, and what am I getting out of it?' Then you're gonna feel a lot better about the whole situation.

And I'm sure that there's gonna be lots of people who are gonna be in the sandwich years, and they'll really look at this and go, 'Yeah, that's me'. And my take-home message is, it is what it is. And if you love your family, you do the best you can with your circumstances. Even if you do get grumpy, even if you do get frustrated and you feel like, 'I can't do this any more', the next day you get up and you just do it anyway.

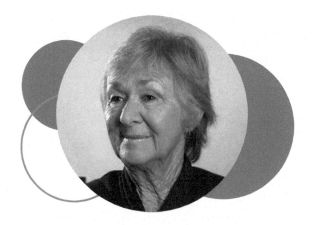

CHAPTER 6

Barbara's story

My name is Barbara and I'm 71 years old. I have had many roles as daughter, wife, mother, grandmother … but 'nana', which I prefer, and great-grandmother and great aunt. I have three sons. One passed away 2 years ago. I have six grandchildren, two surrogate grandchildren, twin boys, and I have two great-nieces and a great-nephew. And I've been very fortunate in always being surrounded with children, which I love. I've always had a very busy life; I worked up until maybe 15 years ago full-time.

I was my mother's oldest daughter and I only had one other sibling, which was a sister, and she became very ill when her two boys were only 13—well, actually they were 12 and 10, and she only lived for 12 months. During the time that she was very ill I spent, because her and her husband lived at the North Coast and I was working full-time, so I would go up every second weekend to see my sister and spend time with her and if she wasn't feeling too good I'd bring the boys back here. And subsequently, because they lost their mother at such an early age I've stepped in and I've been a surrogate mum–aunt, call it what you like but I've always been there for them and they have both lived with myself and my youngest son for certain times during their life … my nephews.

A lot of people have lived here actually over the years. If they haven't got anywhere else to go they come here. So, it's always been a very active, busy household.

Caring for my son

My youngest son broke his neck when he was only 14 and became a quadriplegic so he needed 24/7 care and I was his carer. And it was really good for him with all the activity in the house and people coming and going.

… would have to bath him, brush his hair, clean his teeth, feed him, dress him. I had a lift that you'd pump up and get him in and out of bed, in and out of his chair; he had a motorised wheelchair. When there are a lot of colds and flu around he was very prone to picking those sorts of germs up, which would then go to his chest and pneumonia. When he was, if he was sort of, you know, usually he ended up in hospital but we had the doctor come in every day, twice a day maybe to check in. And I would drag a mattress out into his room and sleep beside his bed so that if he got into difficulties I was right there and he didn't have to call out to me.

When he—was a year in hospital—and well, he was 10 months full-time and then for the last 2 months, because I was working, I would take him to the hospital early in the morning and he'd do his occupational therapy and physiotherapy. Then I'd pick him up after work late in the afternoon and come home and that went on for 2 months until he was ready to be at home full-time. They were very busy times and I often wonder how on earth we got through them, but I did.

Anytime that I was going to do something and that my son wasn't then it meant a lot of organisation because I couldn't just say 'well, I'm going now, I'll see you later'. So I would have to organise somebody to come here. And when I was working, people would come in and out of the house every day.

Caring for my aunt and grandson

An aunt of mine had a stroke, one of my mother's sisters. Her husband had passed away about 7 or 8 years prior to her having her stroke. And they didn't ever have any children. So my mother was her next of kin and then I was the next one, so then she couldn't go home to her home to live any more because she needed 24/7 care. So we had to pack her home up, sort out, sell and discard many, many years of collecting and what have you. But unfortunately she lived on the other side of town so it would take us an hour to get there and another hour home. So our time there was really, really busy and we'd have to get as much done as we possibly could in the hours that I had somebody here looking after my son.

So they were really busy times, as well as, and it was while Ursula was actually in a nursing home after having the stroke that my oldest grandson came to Brisbane because he lived in northern New South Wales with his family, with his mother and he came up here to begin uni. So then started another round of, you know, nana looking after my grandson while he was a uni student. And guiding him as best I could for living and what have you.

Because my grandchildren had always come here for school holidays, the four older ones used to come here every school holidays from when the youngest one was about 3. So they were quite comfortable here, it was their second home. And those times were very demanding because I had four children here and I had a quadriplegic son and everything else that was going on in my life, but somehow it just all happened.

Caring for myself and others

I don't feel a need to slow down just yet. My mind is very, very active and that makes me active physically. I've always been a physically active person. Talking about that too I've got to get back in, I've got this card, which has got about 10 aqua-aerobic classes on it and I've only done a couple of them and I've got to get back into that but it's a bit cold at the moment.

I was mentioning to Margaret the other day that maybe I could go to nursing homes and read to people. I used to read to my aunt a lot when she was in the nursing home. I read to people or because I love animals I'm thinking maybe I could do some work with animals at a shelter.

Reflection—what is old?

It's in your mind thing, as far as I'm concerned. Because I don't put … I've never put an age on me. I've never, I think my mind works just as well as it did when I was 20 or 30. I probably think a little bit more sensibly now if anything.

And I might never have to go into a nursing home. And, you know, my concerns would be, I hope that they would brush my hair and make it look nice of a daytime. And I would hope that if I couldn't dress myself, and they were dressing me, that they would dress me in nice co-ordinated clothing, instead of just throwing anything on. And, you know, just do my body lotions after my shower and just do those nice things.

CHAPTER 7

Wendy's story

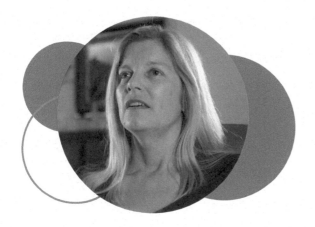

My name's Wendy. I'm a community care manager. I have been a registered nurse for 30 years in aged care. I provide aged care packages to community care clients, home and community care services and private services.

Providing services across areas

We provide services to clients across a large geographical area, from low care, home and community care, domestic shopping assistance, personal care, meal preparation, washing, dressing and medication assistance.

And we also provide extended care packages in the home, almost the equivalent of nursing home care in the home. It can include nursing care, supply of equipment, allied health services such as occupational therapy and physio.

Equipment needed for care

Equipment is provisional on what type of care they receive. So most of them would receive their equipment through the Medical Assistance Scheme (MAS) program where they can apply for equipment such as shower chairs, wheelchairs and sometimes hospital beds.

Safety and maintenance of equipment

We've got to ensure that the equipment is safe for the client and safe for the staff, and we've got to make sure that we have systems in place to ensure that a client is maintaining that equipment safely. Once they come onto the bigger packages of care that maintaining of that equipment becomes the organisation's responsibility.

Some of the problems we do come across really is if the families of the residents won't maintain their equipment safely or if they don't renew the equipment and it becomes unsafe.

Referral and provision of care

With the home and community care and the smaller packages of care, the community aged care or the CAPS, we do not provide allied health services. We would refer to other agencies, so if they needed nursing or physiotherapy or occupational therapy, dietitian, we would refer to either a branch of our own organisation or another organisation. We do work very closely with the other organisations in the area.

For the bigger packages of care, so the extended aged care at home or the extended aged care at home dementia package, we would be expected to provide physio or occupational therapy or dietitian within that bucket of money which the government subsidise us.

Access to services

Access of services can happen quite a number of different ways, so people can access the organisation directly themselves by just calling up, GPs can refer and a lot of them come in after assessment from the aged care assessment team.

Quite often we come across people that have 'crisised' and may be in hospital and that'll be the first they realise that they are entitled to this care.

Working with aged care assessment teams

We work very well with the aged care assessment teams. We have a very close working relationship. They have a large waiting list to go out and assess. So normally what we find is we could maybe put people on some HAC (Home and Community) services, but they are very limited on the amount of hours that we can offer. So normally you would be offering, maybe, 4 hours of domestic assistance, a couple of hours of social support and that's simply not enough for the care needs that these people are presenting with.

We then have to wait for them to be assessed by the aged care assessment team. That can take up to 3 months. We can call up and advise that we have a person in a crisis situation. Also, I work with the hospitals, quite often I would go out on a joint visit with the aged care assessment team.

Managing client waiting lists

Even if they get the okay for a community aged care package, which is the low-level care, we might not have one available. So then we are looking at waiting lists. Not so many waiting lists for the community aged care package, because there is a cost involved and a lot of the elderly people don't want to pay that jumping cost.

But the extended packages … we have massive waiting lists so it's not been unknown to have 20 people on that waiting list. So we normally try and maintain them on a CAPS package until we source an extended aged care at home package for them. Most of them want to stay with our organisation, but we will approach the other organisations in the area to get them the correct care as soon as possible.

Secret to managing gaps in services

The secret of managing the gaps in service is really early assessment of the residents. So part of the problem is that nobody's picked up the changes in a timely manner, so that we may have somebody that … suddenly, I may go out and do an assessment or my co-ordinator and their needs are so high we can't access the bigger packages for them soon enough. We then have to maybe borrow some money from another part of the budget or work with families. Quite a few of the families in my experience have been happy to pay some private services to keep that elderly person in their home. So, for instance, we do a bedding-down service where we'll go along, maybe 8 o'clock in the evening and bed the person down for overnight.

Another way that I've had to deal with it in the past, purely because of financial restrictions, is myself maybe going in and doing some medication assistance and an evening meal on the way home if I've been passing a client's home in the evening on the way home at night. And it's not ideal but we've just really got to juggle a bit like that, but I think the secret really is that early assessment and get the aged care assessment teams out and get people moved on as their needs increase.

Role of volunteers in the community

The other way we've sometimes done it is bringing volunteers on-board, so maybe a volunteer driver. So, they'll get their 4 hours domestic and maybe meal assistance, but we can use a volunteer to take them for their shopping, which costs nothing.

Challenges working in the community

A lot of issues that we deal with is juggling the client and the family wishes with the numerous policies that we need to adhere to and the aged care standards and accreditation guidelines that we've got to adhere to.

One example was an elderly chap—his wife was one of our dementia clients—he had decided to cut the bottom off the shower chair because the lady was not very tall. Unfortunately it became a health and safety risk for our staff and I had to go in and negotiate a solution with him where I got him to agree that we would provide the shower chair. So my staff used the shower chair when we were in and he used his shower chair when we weren't there. We got an independent occupational therapist in to give him some guidance because, obviously, it was a big risk to him and his back.

Importance of policies and procedures

Policies and procedures are very important. We need to look after our residents and our staff and have no injuries, and we need to adhere to the aged care standards, the community care standards. Sometimes the staff find it very difficult to adhere to policies and procedures because they find it very difficult to say no to the families and the relatives out in the homes, because they're working without direct supervision in the homes so some of the residents really try and get a bit extra out of them and they can't say no.

Case study

We had a husband and wife: they both had a CAPs package with ourselves and the wife had persuaded one of my personal carers to wait an extra hour and a half after the session. So she was only supposed to get an hour and the poor worker was waiting two and a half hours and an hour and a half of that was unpaid and she really couldn't say no. She was just such a kind, lovely person. But of course, the next carer that went in insisted she would only stay the hour. And, the lady called me to complain about the worker that would only stay an hour.

A lot of work went on with the personal carers to just explain the repercussions of them not adhering to care plans and not adhering to the policies.

Person-centred care and healthcare reforms

Some of the ideas behind the healthcare reforms are really good. We're looking at care becoming much more person-centred. There is quite a lot of background work that will require to be done with the organisation, in my service in particular. The carers and the clients have been very used to tasks and getting the tasks done. So, for instance, with a consumer-directed package and person-centred care, the client really would be expected to be a bit more independent so when you go to do a domestic service the client would be expected to do as much as they possibly could on their own so you might be saying to them, instead of the way we do it just now, that we do all the vacuuming for them, we might be saying, 'Okay, what can you do? Do you want to do that part and we'll do the parts of the care that you can't do?'

That's a huge mind shift for people, especially for some clients that are paying for a service. So they may think they are paying to have the cleaning done, why should they be doing part of it on their own.

Managing consumer-directed care packages

One of the main problems as a manager that I can foresee I am going to have with the consumer-directed packages is rostering and the finances around that. The client can really decide any day of the week that they've changed their service and they want to have it the next day or not at all or bank the care and have it the following week. That really makes rostering a massive problem.

What some of the other organisations have actually done is make some staff redundant and used brokerage agents to provide their staff so you then phone that brokerage agent and you say, 'Can you give me a carer for 2 hours tomorrow?' and that actually becomes much more cost efficient.

Rewards of being a community manager

It's very rewarding being a manager to clients in the community. I'm very hands on, I do go out and do a lot of those visits and a lot of the complaints I go out and deal with. People really, really want to stay in their communities; that's where they've lived for a number of years. It's very, very important to their families. A lot of the families have promised that they won't put them into care. So it can be hugely challenging but hugely rewarding.

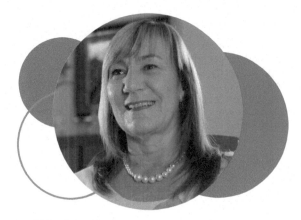

CHAPTER 7

Roseanne's story

My name's Roseanne. I'm a registered nurse. I've worked for 23 years now in the community services with a not-for-profit organisation.

In the community we do a lot of different services to the clients, things like medication administration, medication assistance, we might go and assist with their hygiene, we may be assessing the client to see what capabilities they have and what their care plan might be needed to manage them in their home quite safely, we could be doing chronic wound management or advising the client about other services that are around.

Types of funding for clients

The types of funding that we have to cover those, we would have HACC, which is Home and Community Care, or there may be ... the Department of Veteran Affairs may fund for veterans in the community. There's a large percentage of frail elderly, some young disabled, and there are times when we get funding from the hospital to visit clients after they have been in hospital whether it's because they've had an operation and they've now got an infection or they need some help around the home just till they recuperate enough to continue independently after they've recuperated.

How clients access the services

There are a variety of ways that the clients come into our service. It may be that they know someone down the road who has care and they know to give us a ring and we would receive a call from them and we would work through the process and go out and assess them to identify what their needs are and how we may help them. It may be that the GP might send a referral to us and requesting a specific service like hygiene or wound care or medication administration or assistance, it may be that it's the hospital because the client's been in and had an operation—for example, a total hip replacement—and that the client needs short-term assistance in the home just till they've recuperated and become independent again.

Sometimes it may be a neighbour that rings or it may even be the client's relatives who ring quite concerned that the client isn't managing independently or safely in the home, so that just triggers that we would need to find that the client consents to our visit and then once we get that consent we can go into the home and assess that client and identify the needs and create a care plan with that client.

Refusal of services

Sometimes in the community we have clients who may refuse our services and people around them—the GP or the family or their relatives and their neighbours—may identify that they really are at risk in their home and that they are unsafe or that they're not managing their meals but if the client doesn't consent to us coming in that can be quite an issue because we can't help them if they refuse care.

The registered nurse's day begins ...

A lot of our services start quite early in the morning so from 7, 7.30 in the morning we'll be out visiting clients, the type of things at that time of the day that we would be assisting with would be medication administration, we often do insulin administration, blood sugar levels to monitor the client, to make sure that they're keeping healthy in their home and ensuring that they're eating their meals to manage their diabetes well. We have quite a few dementia clients ... if they are early dementia they may need assistance with their medication rather than administration, so we just ensure that each day we go in they've managed their medications from their Webster packs. So we may lock them away in a box and come in each day and administer those medications so that that way the client is receiving them safely and at the correct time and the correct day.

We also attend clients that have chronic wounds. We would actually assess the whole client to see the type of wound they have, the type of dressing that would be most suitable for that wound and also what the client may be able to afford for the dressing.

Cost of wound care products

The cost of the wound care products is not covered by any of the funding that the clients receive so they have to actually pay for their products and some products can be quite expensive and be more than several dollars a day and it actually is negotiating with the client and showing them the costs of things and helping them to order the products from companies and get them delivered to the home, so that we can have those products there for when we visit each day or every couple of days.

Assessment of the client

If it's a new client to the community, we would come in and do a full assessment of that client and that assessment would include things like their diet and how they are managing cooking their meals to: Can they get to the shops to get their shopping? Can they get to the doctor's surgery for their appointments? Can they manage their medications safely? Are they stockpiling medications? Do we need to initiate a medication review?

We also look at their mobility around their home and the safety in the home so: Are they tripping over cords? Are they tripping over mats? Is there lighting in the bedroom when they get up at night to go to the toilet? Is there light outside the front door so that if a stranger comes to the door they can answer the door safely? Can they get out in case of a fire? We do a full assessment, not just on their health needs but on how they're managing in the community and what sort of services may help them to get out. Some clients can be quite isolated in their home because they can't get down the stairs or because they're incontinent and they don't want to go out because they're conscious of their continence problems.

So really, a full assessment of the client can make a huge difference to identify what's going to help them to be as independent as possible, to stay in their home for as long as possible … just to be part of the community again and not be isolated in a home where they can become depressed and not eat and become frail and end up in hospital and maybe in care before they really need to be.

Documentation as a reference point

A large portion of our day is taken up with documentation, and documentation is extremely important. There are a lot of staff who feel that it's overwhelming. But it's really, really important to document what you do: it's a legal document, it's a record of what's been happening with the client on a day-to-day basis and it really is a reference point for other staff who see that client to know exactly what's been happening. So even if you've never met the client, everything should be in the documents.

We're often assessing clients and then writing care plans so that we can delegate the care to our personal care workers, to enrolled nurses and endorsed enrolled nurses, and it's really important that if we have assessed the client well and identified exactly what they need then the care plan should be clear for those other care workers. They also need to know when they should ring the nurse because that can be a bit confusing for care workers. What's urgent? What's not? When should I call the nurse to say there's a problem in this home?

Care planning and review

I think it's really important with our care plans too, that we be clear to the care worker what the client is still able to do, so that can be quite an important part of care plans in the community.

Then there's assessments and reviews; every client needs to be reviewed. The amount of times you do reviews will depend on the client's condition. There's a lot of clinical decision-making on a day-to-day basis about: When do we set that next review? When would we need to step in and do the care instead of the care worker? Also, all the decision-making around the delegation: Is it appropriate for the client? Is the care worker capable of that particular task that you are trying to do?

Delegation of care and decision-making

We do a lot of delegation of care to unregulated staff and enrolled nurses.

Some of the clients can be unchanging and stable for some months and that may be appropriate then to delegate care workers to do some of the tasks in that home, but if I had a chronic wound or some clinical care that I was doing then I wouldn't be delegating those tasks to care workers or enrolled nurses. The decision-making can sometimes sound quite complex, but it often comes back to: Is it appropriate for the client? Is it appropriate for the care worker or the enrolled nurse? And what's the legislation behind, maybe, the medications and any other task that you are doing in the home?

So it may seem like a great cost-saving exercise to send a care worker out to assist a client with medications. Is this safe to do? And if in doubt always send the registered nurse. It really is important to think back to what is going to be the safest for this client and what's going to work best.

Policies and procedures

Policies and procedures within an organisation, I found, are very good at giving us clear guidelines on how to interpret the legislation that's out there and on a day-to-day basis how we need to see the clients, how we need to interact with other services and how we to need to manage the care under the funding in a safe manner and also to do with our registration.

Some of the policies and procedures may be a little bit broad so there's still some decision-making left to the registered nurse, but usually you can refer to a manager or contact someone that may have some guidance for you if that was a problem.

Future of consumer-directed care

In the future, there's a possibility of having consumer-directed packages. With those packages the client will be having a lot more control over how their funding is spent on the care that is coming into the home.

If a client was on insulin then I really need to get there early in the morning before breakfast to give that client insulin. But if a client is having hygiene assistance then I may not need to go until later in the day. With the consumer packages it may be that the client decides that they want a 7.30 visit for their hygiene assistance and their personal carer, and that would actually mean then, who's going to be around to do the insulin. So I think that it could be quite a bit of negotiating with clients to really meet their expectations.

Rostering and really knowing how much care or how many client hours you are going to have each day is going to be quite tricky. It's very hard to be everywhere at the same time.

Meeting client expectations: case study

We did have a client in the community … very, very elderly lady whose daughter cared for her in the home. The client was extremely frail and bedridden and we were going in each day to assist her with her hygiene and personal care. The daughter—having looked after the mother for so long—was very, very particular about everything that was done for the mother. If it was a new care worker or if you tried to do something different, the daughter actually got quite angry and would be quite difficult to deal with.

We actually got extra funding to send the nurse and really made it so that the nurse went in each day and parts of the care were done by the daughter and other parts of the care were done by the nurse. It seemed that that allayed the anxieties of the relative, the daughter that was the carer, and it also meant that the registered nurses were a little bit more able to negotiate with that relative on a day-to-day basis, how to care for the mother and we managed to keep the client in the community with her daughter.

But it was very hard for the nurses on a day-to-day basis to really meet the daughter's expectations with timeframes and we had to be there right on 11 and we had to do everything precisely so. But if you were away on leave or if you were on holidays then another care nurse would go in and she'd get anxious because it was a new person and maybe they wanted to change the routine again. So that was quite complex and quite difficult, and it was about keeping the daughter's anxieties at bay but still managing to look after the mother.

Finding optimal solutions for clients in the community

After 23 years nursing in the community, I've really had a lot of satisfaction from the responses I get from the clients when you come into their homes. Most of them are so happy to see you and they're so pleased that someone is actually there listening to them and being able to assist them to work their way through an amazing amount of complex health systems.

It's really a matter of the explanations that you give the clients, and the care is only a very small part, the tasks are a small part, there's a lot of education to do, there's a lot of explanations to do, there's a lot of referrals to do and, obviously, the documentation that relates to all their care.

It's really about the client. Do they want to stay in their home or are they looking at going into care? What's going to be the best solution for that person in their home so that they can live a quality, fulfilling life? And the responses we get from the majority of them is that, 'Thank you for helping', 'I am so pleased you came', 'That makes it clearer' or 'Wow! We stayed here much longer!'

We even have palliative clients in the community quite often and the fact that that person can die at home in peace with the family around or they may choose to go to hospital but whatever they choose we can help them down that road and help the way to be smooth. So, yeah, it's very satisfying and the clients are able to voice their concerns of where they want to be and how they want to live their life and I think we are very privileged to go into their homes and be invited in to help them to do … to really be independent and to stay safe as long as they want to.

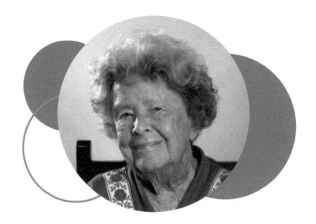

CHAPTER 7

Barbara's story

My name is Barbara. I'm 91 years old. I live by myself in my house, which is three bedrooms, about 10 steps up the back and six in the front on 24 perches. I have a lot of garden which I love doing.

Why is it important for you to live in your own home?

Independence. I love being independent, I love being on my own, I don't need people around me and it's mine!

After my second daughter married about 50 years ago, I've been on my own.

It's good, independence. You don't have to worry about anyone else and you can please yourself.

I just get out of bed and get breakfast, have a shower, make my bed, tidy the house, do a little bit of weeding in the garden each day. I do crosswords, I read.

I'm perfectly happy living alone, always have been.

What can you no longer do for yourself?

I can't climb up and clean my windows. I don't mow the lawn any more and I can't work in the garden like I used to. I used to work for hours in the garden, so you've just got to do a little bit at a time, when you can, which is very frustrating actually.

I can't climb up on chairs to fix curtains or clean windows, just as long as I can do it from the floor it's okay. But I don't climb up on chairs any more. <laughs>

What help do you get to stay at home?

I have a lady who comes once a fortnight to do the floors and I have a mower man now.

To go shopping, my daughter takes me and I do all my own shopping. She insists on taking me otherwise I would get a cab. They issued me with … the OT people issued me with a walking stick, but it's beneath me to use a walking stick. <laughs> I could not feel happy walking around with a walking stick. So I get a trolley and that's my walking stick.

I have a physio—comes once a week—and I have occupational therapy—sees me about once every 6 months—and that's it.

What does the physiotherapist do?

Because of my back and also I've got calcium deposits on my hip, which causes a bit of pain, and she comes and shifts the things around and try to get rid of it for a couple of hours.

What does the occupational therapist do?

She only comes about once every 6 months and she gets me to draw certain designs and count backwards in 7s from a hundred. And, she gives me three words to remember and then asks me what they were about 10 minutes later to see if I still remember.

The Vet Affairs ordered it, because I'm under Vet Affairs. They're very good. The Vet Affairs look after you very well.

What is your health like?

I've had my gall bladder out … about 4 years ago and then I had to go back in because there was a stone stuck in the bile duct, so that was within a week of the other operation.

I've had a couple of cancers taken out. I've had my tonsils out. <laughs>

I'm very healthy! Yes, I've been very fortunate.

I take a blood pressure tablet and a Fosamax, which is for the bones.

Do you ever get frightened or feel isolated living alone?

No, no, I don't. I don't even think about it.

I'm not a people person so I'm quite okay on my own. I don't need people around me.

Barbara was burgled three times over the last couple of years

Oh well, they were a bit sneaky. I was sitting watching TV in the lounge and they came in through our bedroom window and he took my money, my purse with my money and all your credit cards and personal stuff you have in there. And, what annoyed me most about it is he went under the house and got the ladder to climb up into the bedroom and then he didn't even have the decency to put the ladder back.

I rang the police and they came over and, but, there's not much they can do about it. Then about a year later I had another fella that came in the same way, I don't know how he got in because he didn't use the ladder, but he took my purse all the same. And then, I had, my next-door neighbour could look into my kitchen from her balcony and she came into me, in the afternoon and she said, 'you had a visit from your grandson today?' and I said, 'no' and she said, 'well, there was a man in your kitchen!' So he came in through the back door and he was looking around my kitchen apparently and I'm sitting in the lounge room and then he goes off up the road and he's gonna hide. So after that I thought three strikes and I got security all around the house. So I'm all locked in, in jail now so nobody can get in.

Barbara now has a VitalCall system

You gotta wear this thing around your neck, you know, with the button there. I suppose it does make you safe, you've got to check with them once a month. One day I dropped a spot of gravy on it and I went to wipe it off and it BOOO everything … and everything went off! <laughs> And I had to apologise for doing it, you know, unnecessarily.

You can stand in my kitchen, which is away from where the VitalCall is, and talk to them. It reaches quite a while and they said even if you're downstairs and it goes off they may not be able to talk to you but they will send someone or they'll get in touch with Barb, or they'll send somebody out to see that you're okay. I suppose it is handy but you've got to feel a bit of a dill with this thing around your neck all the time.

Would you ever consider going into a nursing home?

I would hate it! Absolutely hate it! I could not bear the lack of privacy, the lack of freedom to do what I want, when I want, how I want. And I would hate not being able to make myself some Promite and onion sandwiches. <laughs> I eat a lot of onions, I have eaten a lot of onions and I reckon that's why I've been so healthy all my life. We used to eat them like apples when we kids.

What do you attribute to staying fairly healthy, active and independent?

I think, basically, genes have got a lot to do with it, but I've never smoked and I've never drank. I'll have an occasional red wine, very occasional, I don't go out with bad men <laughs> and that's about it. I've just lived an active life and I think that just keeps you going.

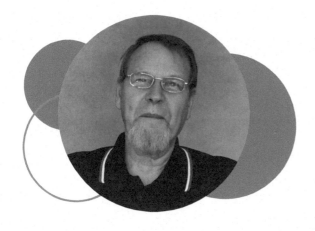

CHAPTER 8

Robert's story

My name is Robert. I'm 66 years old.

My story

I have learned to live with chronic back pain out of necessity. How it happened: I was a member of the Harley Davidson Club Amsterdam, and during the summer months we would spruce up our bikes and we would go and tour around, we would stop at a nice little restaurant, or one of the famous coffee shops, have hash cake and an iced coffee, and then we would continue through the countryside. On one of those days we did exactly that, had done that before, and out of nowhere a car just swiped, 'pfoom', swiped me right off my bike, the next thing I know is I'm strapped into a stretcher.

I was strapped down with leather belts, like I didn't know what on earth … that was all they had in those days, they didn't have all the modern equipment, but that in hindsight was to stop me from moving about.

Went in hospital, they did some tests and they … I was in traction for a while, and I was told that I had three fractured vertebrae, lumbar vertebrae, and severe damage to the cartilage. And after several visits and specialists come around, they said, 'We might be able to help you by having an operation where we remove all the bits and pieces, and we will fuse the two vertebrae together. We wait for them to heal first, then we fuse them together, and that will reduce mobility in the lumbar region, but it will also take away the risk and the pain. You'll be a centimetre shorter'. That's enough for me to say, 'No thank you very much'.

And so I was 3 months out of action, and I used crutches, but regretfully I ended up not using them as I should, because being young and rebellious you think you can do without. I'm now paying the price for that.

In hindsight the advice that I'd been given was probably … I should have listened to that. I remember one of the old nurses coming up to me and said to keep the weight off for as long as possible, and really take those 3 months to be very careful. But as a young person, you don't like walking around on crutches and that was just not done. As an older person now, I wish I had listened to her because it might have made a big difference. As the operation is concerned, I'm still doubtful whether I would have made the right decision then, or the wrong decision by not proceeding with it, but that's something that you just have to accept, because that cannot be undone.

Managing my pain

How do I manage my pain? Well, a lot of it was trial and error. One of the main things I find now as my body is getting older, I am far more aware not to perform acute movements. So if someone were to call my name, rather than just swing your head around and have a look, I turn around completely around my axis so as not to twist my spine. And one of the other things is wherever I sit I make sure there are seats that have armrests so I can get up without, you know, hurting myself. And one of the other things I find I'm using, like Panadol Osteo, or different things. I avoid lifting things, and in general a lot of the things I used to do out of habit I just had to stop, which makes it sometimes unpleasant.

One of the problems also I found was that when you talk to the doctor, and they also suggest, 'Oh, we'll have you see a specialist'. And then you have to report the whole thing over and over again. I know what is wrong with me, and I know it can't be fixed any more. So that after a while I just gave up, and I'm quite happy sort of going to the chemist and see what they have, and what I can try, and it means I don't have to go back to make an appointment, to see a doctor again, and then get a prescription for something that's doing the same thing that I can just do … get from the chemist.

Living with this has affected my lifestyle a lot. One of the sad things is that when family comes around, and the kids are around, and some of the toddlers they come out and they want to be picked up, I can't do it; I just refuse to do it because I know the consequences.

It's hard to have to explain over, and over, and over, and that is really annoying. So you withdraw a little bit, so you end up sitting on the sideline so you don't get too involved. When my family goes tenpin bowling, I sit on the sideline because I just can't do it any more. And strangers see me there, sitting there on the side, thinking, 'Oh, this man doesn't even want to participate with family outings', but that's not what it is. It's just being self-aware to make very, very sure that I don't hurt myself unnecessarily.

My hobby used to be motorbikes and sailing, the sailing has gone by the way, I just cannot get in and out, or I'm just not agile enough any more, and the bending and jumping around is just too dangerous for me to do.

As an older person, it's frustrating to notice that the opinion of people are if you're not quick enough out of the way, and things like that, and people don't know your situation, that makes it not embarrassing, but it makes it frustrating, because there is a reason why I cannot just get up and go, and there is a reason I find it hard to get in those pokey little modern cars, or get out of them again.

What I'm doing differently now that I'm older, being more aware, when you're younger your body tends to be more forgiving, and also being a bit of a rebel you think you'll be all right, and it doesn't apply to you. Well, I have been wearing a brace now for a long time that I could omit when I was younger. I can … there are days I cannot actually sit without the brace on, which is … it's annoying, and it also limits your movement a lot.

Experiences with healthcare professionals

When I was younger talking to doctors, I tended to listen: they were fast in their explanations, and it was all a matter of fact. Now, however, I find it very hard to have to listen to them, because I have been living with this for quite a long time now. They ask you often, 'Explain the pain level'. How do you explain pain on a level, points? That is rather annoying. I mean, pain is different for a lot of people, and at times I feel like saying to them, 'It's like pulling my teeth out with the pliers, eating hot soup and cold ice cream at the same time', that's the type of feeling you get. And also having to listen that there might now be new systems and new technology, and I don't want to take any risks any more. Also when I'm confronted by a doctor that is just graduated, it's very hard. I've been living with this for a long time, and it's very hard to make them understand I'm not interested in any new ideas any more, I'm quite happy to continue and manage it myself this way.

I think at times the medical profession, as you are an older person or an older patient, they tend to take it rather personal if you try to offer a different opinion, or sometimes contradict them. And on the other side, the medical profession tends to talk to you as if you do not know your own body, and they know best, and that is very frustrating to have to put up with. So it's one of the reasons I've just stopped going to surgeries, and it's one of the reasons that I just keep doing what I'm doing now.

For older people I definitely would recommend trying out different things, don't stay beholden to your doctor however wrong that might sound at the moment, but a lot of those guys haven't tried much themselves really, let's be honest.

When you're an older person you don't see yourself as old, it's only younger persons that see you as an older person. See, that's … so that's a constant battle. So you go to a doctor that is only 30 years old, and he's telling you things, and you know you've already done it or tried it, but to him it's new, and to you it's old hat, and he takes it as a personal affront that you say, 'Well, sorry, mate, but doesn't work'. So it doesn't go down very well.

CHAPTER 8

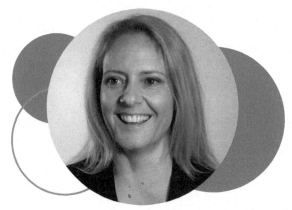

Leonie's story

Hi, my name is Leonie and I am a naturopath. I studied for 3 years to become a naturopath. There is a lot of science studying to be a naturopath.

Naturopathy and nutrition

Natural therapists can work in a number of places. Massage therapists, for example, can work from home or in massage therapy clinics, acupuncturists can do the same setting up a private practice or working from their own clinic and naturopaths can actually work from their own clinic or in chiropractic offices or in health food shops.

Nutrition is a major part of natural medicine and, in particular, naturopathy. A naturopath will spend a lot of time going through the diet and actually looking at what a person eats, what they have for breakfast, lunch and dinner. We work to help people balance their blood sugar levels by making little changes to their diet, promoting healthy eating, eating more vegetables and eating whole foods, real foods, because a lot of people nowadays are eating packaged and processed or refined foods and have really lost their way. They are confused by what information is out there in the media, they are confused about whether something is healthy or not healthy for them so in naturopathy we work to help re-educate people and take them back to basics of good eating, wholesome eating and real foods.

We start from babies, and in fact before babies, so we have pregnant women or couples that are looking to start a family and then from the very beginning of life, from the newborn baby and advice on what the mother should be eating during lactation so that she gets the best promotion of good milk flow and all the way through the life stages, so introducing solid food, something that a naturopath can do is help a parent choose the foods that are best to start with the baby and that way they can be mindful of any allergies or sensitivities to food that may show up. Working all the way through the age groups, up through teenagers, through menopause and then into the older age groups as well.

Ageing and naturopathy

Many people, as they age, come to see natural therapists and naturopaths. The men will come often for prostate problems so they may have been diagnosed with an inflamed prostate or just changes in urinary function and so there are a lot of things that a naturopath can do to actually help to promote a good flow of urine and natural anti-inflammatories to promote good health.

The women often come because they are worried about the man; to be honest with you, many women are more proactive than men I find in medicine and in natural medicine. But often they come because after menopause some women experience hypertension or high blood pressure, as do the men, or they tend to start to notice changes in their gastrointestinal functions. Many men and women are noticing that they become more bloated than they used to and they are starting to see different foods that are causing bloating.

One of the things that they can do in naturopathy is come to us and we help them look at different foods and make different choices, so it is about replacing foods rather than taking things away. It is about replacing them with other options that alleviate the gastrointestinal issues.

Some people come in and they actually have cardiovascular conditions such as hypertension or high blood pressure and they may have been put on medication but they are really quite keen to reduce the medication. So working in conjunction with a GP you can actually promote a different lifestyle and different food choices and some supplements. Simple supplementation such as … magnesium is a natural mineral that will help to reduce the pressure in the arteries, so it is a natural muscle relaxant. We can use vitamin C and bioflavonoids to promote healthy arteries, vitamin E to slightly thin the blood and fish oils to promote good blood flow as well. Working in conjunction with the GP they can then actually, hopefully, reduce the amount of medications that they are on because they are making good changes in their diet.

The older person and the naturopath

I have noticed a lot more older people are starting to come in to ask advice now. They still go to their GP and then they come to us because they know that there is something missing. Many of them share stories of when they were growing up and they used to eat differently, and, you know, they share stories of their grandparents, for example, and how the grandmother used to say, 'eat your vegetables and eat this herb' because this herb was the particular thing that would keep them flu-free during the winter and so they come back for that sort of information. I find they talk to me and they remember what they used to do.

Often older clients will come in and they will share their experiences that they have with their GPs and what they are looking for is someone who will spend more time with them and actually talk to them more about their diet and their lifestyle and unfortunately, due to time restraints and also due to their training, a GP doesn't go through diet and lifestyle with them so much, so they come to us and they will look for that sort of information.

Many people, when they come in, share their experiences of how they are ageing and many of them don't feel older until something is going wrong with their body or something is changing and then that is when they notice what age they actually are. So they come to a naturopath and we actually work with them to help to make simple changes in their life that can promote energy and promote better health and to promote them feeling better within themselves.

So we might work with diet and lifestyle, we might work with encouraging them to take up a hobby that they have never done or even some studies just to keep them active. A lot of people that come in, as they age, they share that they may be nervous about things like dementia or memory changes and I find for most of them that are talking about it, they actually have a history of memory changes or dementia in the family and so that is where their nerves come from. I work with lifestyle techniques so promoting using their brains, you know, reading and doing quizzes and puzzles, the general things that you would imagine, but also natural remedies to promote good brain function. There are herbs like ginkgo and bacopa which is known as brahmi. Vitamin E is another thing that we can use and that is a naturopath's version of an aspirin as it thins the blood, so it thins the blood and also it is an antioxidant so it promotes good brain health and good cell health.

Another thing that naturopaths will do is we chat to people. I find that a lot of people come in and they really haven't had someone to chat to in quite some time. Perhaps they have lost a partner or quite often the family won't live quite close by so they will come to the naturopath, and because we spend an hour with them, it is a great opportunity to actually chat. I also work in a health food shop and many people come in and it's a quick thing that they want. They will come in for one supplement and spend 20 to 30 minutes chatting to you about their experiences and their life.

One of the simplest things that I recommend for people to do when they age is to continue to drink water or to remember to drink water because so many people are drinking tea and coffee and not water. Unfortunately, they are getting mixed information about that; they are being told that tea and coffee is water but tea and coffee is not water, they generally work as a diuretic in the body making the loss of fluids rather than promoting the retention of fluids or hydrating the cells. I have noticed when people drink water their brain function is better, their concentration levels are better and generally they feel better within themselves. Also it improves their taste so drinking water will improve that dry mouth that a lot of people get, so less salt needed on their food, more water: simple.

My uncle, I remember many years ago he was at home and the following day he went into hospital but I remember visiting him and he had dementia and he didn't really recognise me and was very confused. He'd been drinking a lot of tea, a lot of cups of tea that day and really, his memory was quite poor. Anyway, the next day he was in hospital and by the time I got there to see him, it was quite interesting because they'd had him on fluids all day and when I got there he greeted me. It was, 'hello, Leonie' and he was so lucid he asked me so many questions and chatted away to me. The only difference that had happened was that he had been given fluids and had been hydrated so his memory was back and he was feeling good, he was saying, 'What am I doing in this place?'

The aged care setting and the naturopath

Naturopaths can work with people in aged care. It is a great opportunity for a naturopath to go in and work to advise on different foods that can be incorporated into aged care.

One of the sadder stories I heard was through a colleague who was working in a health food shop and actually it makes me upset. She had a woman come in who was in aged care and she said it was a beautiful facility, wonderful carers, wonderful nurses there and the staff were just beautiful. She said it was a lovely place but what she was missing were vegetables. For this particular lady, my colleague actually recommended some super foods, so this woman, and she was in her eighties, really missing vegetables but so willing to do anything. She had like a sink and she could have a blender in her room so she was making herself smoothies and adding super foods to her smoothies and she added chia seeds and things like Vital Greens or your green super foods just to add to it. It is not really a vegetable but it is the nutrients from vegetables; that was what she was missing.

You know, from my perspective, if I could get into aged care facilities and actually work to promote more use of vegetables, fresh veggies for people, because that is what they grew up on, I think that would make a huge difference to their health and their wellbeing. Many older people grew up with veggie gardens and so, you know, perhaps that is something that could be incorporated into aged care facilities is that they start growing vegetable gardens. I think most people could do with a veggie garden nowadays but perhaps that is one way of getting more vegetables, and getting people, you know, the people that are active can get out there and work in the garden, they love it and it is that sense of wellbeing, that sense of purpose plus they are growing food that they get to eat.

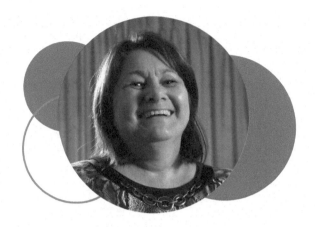

CHAPTER 8

Judy's story

Hi, I'm Judy McCrow. I'm from a nursing background. I'm a registered nurse.

Delirium and dementia

So what is delirium? It's what they call an acute confusional state. So there is an acute change in cognition as opposed to dementia which is a gradual decline in cognition or ability to think their memories so there's lots of different changes that occur.

The significance with delirium is that it's potentially a reversible disorder even if it's in someone who's already got a dementia. Dementia is probably the biggest risk factor for delirium. So we often see delirium superimposed on dementia on someone in hospital; however, what you often hear is the behaviour is just because their dementia got worse when they're in hospital when realistically there's probably some underlying cause for this change in behaviour that needs to be assessed.

The shorter a duration of delirium, the better outcomes there are for a patient. So potentially a patient with delirium can actually have increased risks of falls, pressure injuries, immobility, decrease in functional decline leading to residential aged care environment. So a lot of these people, especially if they've come in with an underlying dementia and develop a delirium, they might've come from home, but they might have to go back to a residential aged care facility. Whereas if this delirium is found and treated, it's potentially reversible, so the sooner it's found and treated the better the outcomes there are for the person.

Delirium and depression

The other important thing to notice is, when you talk about delirium dementias, they talk about the three Ds which is delirium, dementia and depression. For example, one type of delirium is a hypoactive type of delirium where the person's sitting in the chair and doesn't want to do anything and that's often misdiagnosed as depression and the problem being is they'll start getting treated for depression but the cause of delirium is never found.

So potentially they could have a UTI that by the time it's found it's actually a rip-roaring sepsis and the person's likely to die because they've been treated as a depression because they look like depression. So if we're able to identify the delirium and to make the difference—the differential diagnosis—that again will have different outcomes for the people.

When I see someone with hypoactive delirium, one of the things you can actually do is continue asking the same question. If it's a delirium they probably won't be able to answer the question at any stage, whereas if it's depression eventually they will give you an appropriate answer. Not always working, but it's a simple strategy to try.

Cognitive impairment

So now I'll just actually talk about cognitive impairment as a whole so it's not just about delirium or just about dementia or delirium superimposed on dementia, it's about cognitive impairment. So if we just think of the group of people together in one group … so what actually happens now is they're not getting recognised when they come into the facility. So there's lots of problems if they're not getting recognised and one of it is especially if they've come in with a cognitive impairment, whether it's pre-existing or a new presentation of it, is they're unable to ask questions so they're often not eating very well, they're not drinking very well, they can't get re-orientated into the different environment, so they don't know where the toilet is.

So these people become what they call 'incontinent' in hospital, so they go home wearing incontinence pants when they came in fully continent. It's probably because of the management strategies that have been implemented when they were in hospital. So the key initially is to recognise cognitive impairment whether it's pre-existing or a new episode of it.

So we need to have systems in place where cognitive impairment is identified, whether it's pre-existing or it's a new diagnosis, so appropriate management strategies can be implemented.

There needs to be a system-wide approach to caring for people with cognitive impairment. So I'm probably talking a lot more about the acute care sector but the same has to go within the residential aged care facilities. Both acute care and residential aged care facilities have standards in place that govern their practice and they're accredited against these standards.

So, at the moment, cognitive impairment is not actually covered in all those standards. So the facilities actually have to think more broadly about what they can implement to actually improve practice and management for these people when they come into either hospital or residential aged care environments.

So, systems are the first thing, the other thing is staff training. At the moment, people have lots of training to do with lots of things when they come into the health care facility whether they're nurses or doctors but cognitive impairment is just a small bit of undergraduate training.

So skills and training need to be implemented into facilities if we want people to provide best practice. So it's not because nurses or doctors don't want to do the right thing, it's because they don't know how to do the right thing. And it's about simple strategy so it's not about highfalutin' medications or treatment management plans for these people. It's about simple best practice, how to manage someone when they've got behavioural disturbances.

So don't think about the behaviour itself and think that we have to give them psychographics, for example, to manage the behaviour. There's other simple strategies that we can do before we go to psychotropic therapy and that's something that's still commonly practised, especially in acute care sectors and it's because the nurses don't know anything differently.

Managing cognitive impairment and delirium

So, ideally, when someone comes into hospital, an older person, so even with prior cognitive impairment or at risk of developing delirium when they're in hospital, the best practice would be to actually identify that change in behaviour or the cognition at an early stage and continue to monitor it throughout their hospitalisation. Because, especially if they've come in with a delirium, they might look like they've resolved but because of the nature of the disorder—it could be fluctuating—it could reappear in a day's time or something. So we need to continually monitor that.

So the first thing is to recognise the behaviour and then have a pathway to follow so there's appropriate treatment. For delirium, currently most treatment that I see in acute care facilities is actually drug therapy and ideally we shouldn't actually have to go that far. If we can recognise it early, then we can actually stop the aggressive behaviours that are a consequence of the delirium. So if we can find and treat the cause early, that's the first-line management strategy for any delirium so it's to find and treat the cause. Delirium by nature and by the DSM standards is actually caused by some medical problem.

Having said that, it could be multi-factorial, so especially in intensive care environments where delirium is really prevalent it is hard to treat. In the medical wards I actually find a lot of it is like simple constipation or some medications that they might be on. So they're the simple strategies we need to look at, because if it is constipation or potentially a UTI, if they've come in from a residential aged care facility, they're things we can actually find quite easily. And I've actually found full resolution of symptoms of delirium simply by treating the constipation, or in some cases managing the pain with Panadol.

So, people, if they've come in with pre-existing cognitive impairment, it's hard to assess if they've got pain and they're certainly not going to tell you that they've got pain. So if we think about when their behaviours change, it might be a needs-driven behaviour, so it could be something as simple as pains, so by giving them simple analgesic we might curb the behaviour.

So if you try to think about yourself … if you've got pain, you do tend to become agitated yourself so it's no different if people with cognitive impairment except they can't tell you that they've got the pain.

The carer role

So also another important strategy for people with cognitive impairment is to involve the carers, especially when they first come into the facility, because the person with dementia or delirium or delirium superimposed on dementia is often unable to give you a full or accurate history. So you might actually talk to them and they tell you that they are managing at home and they take their medications and they do all their own shopping when realistically they're probably not. So you need to involve carers to actually get a really, really good history, so that's the key when people first come in to the facility; just to get a history from the carer.

The other thing is, actually, to involve carers in the management of people in hospital as much as possible so if they're able to get them to sit there during meal times and help with meals or stay in the evening until the person is going to sleep.

The other thing carers can be involved in is actually emergency response procedures. So, if carers are aware, if they've come in to visit their relative and for some reason the behaviour's quite bizarre or quite different to what they're used to, then they need to know that they can escalate and call someone for help or actually call an emergency.

Case study

I did a recent night shift where a lady actually came in from a residential aged care facility, she had a known dementia and she had a delirium superimposed on the dementia. And good practice, they actually found it was a UTI. So that … they had found the cause of the delirium and they were treating it; however, the antibiotics actually hadn't started to kick in so she still had some agitated behaviours.

Being at night time, this was a real concern to the nursing staff so she was 'specialed', so she had a nurse special within the ward area. The nurse actually called for assistance because the lady was starting to get increasingly agitated. So I went in there and I was followed closely behind with the team leader. And the team leader, her immediate response was, 'What medications can we give this lady for this agitation?' And, I actually asked the nurse like, 'Why do you want to give this lady some medication?' And the answer was, 'Because she is agitated'.

I actually said to hold back on the medication so let's try some other principles, let's turn the lights on to start to try and actually re-orientate this lady to the environment a little bit. Let's give her a drink, let's try and distract her by looking at pictures or magazines. The lady settled quite quickly by just turning the lights on so she probably was just a bit frightened in a different environment that she didn't know.

The nurse that was actually 'specialing' this lady overnight continued to do this throughout the night and she needed no psychotropic therapies.

So if we can actually not give it, it's much better for the patient. Once you start giving the psychotropics and getting into that cycle of psychotropic therapy that's when they stay in bed, that's when they have the functional decline and that's when they need to go to residential aged care rather than to go back to their home environment.

Summary

So, in summary, there's three strategies that we need to implement to improve practice for people with cognitive impairment when they come into residential aged care facilities and also in acute care. So the first strategy or mechanism in place needs to be a systems-wide approach. So we need to make sure there's policies and procedures in place. Clinical pathways are being used, evidence-based practice is being implemented and there's monitoring of these practices, and policies and procedures are continually updated. So that's from a systems-wide point of view.

The next thing is staff education and training so we need to make sure our staff are educated and trained into recognising cognitive impairment plus best practice for management of people with cognitive impairment.

And the next thing is partnering with carers and consumers. So we need to involve carers in the management and also obtaining histories from people when they come into hospital and again into residential aged care facility.

So they're the three main strategies that need to be implemented by residential aged care facilities and acute care facilities to provide optimal management strategies for people with cognitive impairment involving dementia, delirium, and delirium when it's superimposed on dementia and even people when they come in with mild cognitive impairment.

I guess the main things to think about, especially from a nursing point of view, and it doesn't matter if it's a registered nurse, an AIN or enrolled nurse, I always try to educate people about back-to-basic care. So think about constipation, think about potential UTIs as being a cause of the change in behaviours, think about pain. It's quite often these simple strategies that actually work and we, as nurses, can do those strategies without involving medical intervention.

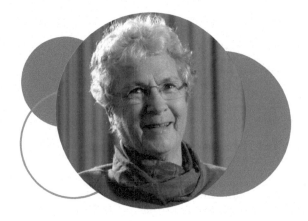

CHAPTER 9

Maureen's story

I'm Maureen Brady, and I'm now 74 years of age.

I always thought high maintenance meant that I'd be having massages and my hair done and my facials. High maintenance, however … for myself, became doctors' appointments. I was diagnosed with breast cancer. So that sort of made me realise that some of this must be about me.

Some of this must be about me

When I was first diagnosed, John—my husband—was very unaccepting. He didn't want to know, that couldn't be happening because I was all about him, and that happens. So I had to just sort of initially go through it by myself, and at the same time make provision for him in my life.

So over the years, I am now out of the other end of my cancer, and very, very happy to be so, and feeling a sense of … that yes, I have conquered that, I've come through, I've done everything I've been told to do.

Now, as perhaps a control freak, I don't know, but I've always been in charge of my children, my mother's care, my brother died along the way with his cancer. So going through all those, you adjust what your role is, it's changing all the time. And you have to be prepared to do that, because the minute you start to fight that, or to want to cling to the old ways, the more stress it puts on yourself, and therefore it doesn't do you any good, and if you're no good to yourself, you are no good to those that you are caring for.

The things of life

Have somewhere to go every day, even if it's for a little walk to communicate with other people, to see something. An older person walking their dog, an older couple walking along supporting each other, they're the things of life, and they're the things that keep you—on a day-to-day basis—keep you positive and thinking away from yourself with your health problems. That can be really a down thing, because if you're focused on only that, but if you look after yourself, and without being paranoid, but just general wellbeing—looking at things like what you eat and how much red wine you have of an evening—that's always helpful. Good for the heart, good for the spirits.

So it's about being positive and, as I say, back to my mother, she was a very strong woman, and I think genetically I got that from her, but it's always been the family that got me through the first time; it got me through the cancer.

Facing the advanced health directive

Recently when John's last hospitalisation … we had the situation where the end-of-life paperwork had to be done. I've had the forms for that, advanced directive, I've had the forms in a drawer for quite some time. I've never been able to fill it in. When we came to the need that it must be done, after this recent hospitalisation, I had to get my daughter to do it, my nurse daughter who knows all about it. I couldn't do that. So, mmm.

Death holds no fear

When I get into that area, where that's inevitable <upset> … but anyway, not my call, and we shall see, but I don't dwell on it. It's just those momentary things.

My brother had cancer, 5-year battle, and I sat with him while he died. I sat with my mother while she died, physically sat there and talked them through it. Now because of that, it has no fear for me personally. And I don't fear for John, we're Catholic, he's been anointed and all those things. It's just the practical side of things, and I don't dwell on it but it is there.

It's easy for me to sit here fit and healthy to say that, but I have been down the other roads, and to come out the other end has been the support of friends and family. But it has also been a lot of educating yourself: if you really want to do it, go ahead, find a way, find a way to do it.

CHAPTER 9

Shirley's story

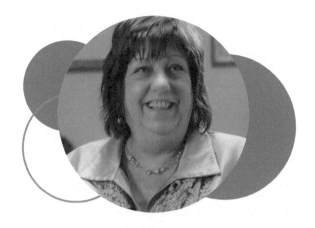

I've been a director of nursing in aged care since 1996. I've worked for for-profits, not-for-profits and government aged care facilities.

Philosophy of customers

During the time that I've been in this position, I've noticed a huge change in the focus of the way people's care deliveries are delivered. The expectations of our customers that we call them now instead of them being our residents, and I believe that it's an excellent improvement in the way that we deliver care. And going forward into the future, it will be the way care will have to be delivered. Our customers are much more aware of their rights and they have high expectations of the type of care that they expect when they're in an aged care facility.

So that's made an enormous difference in the way that we deliver care. Because we also speak about looking at what's positive about the resident rather than the deficits that they have. So, for instance, if someone's had a stroke and they've got a left-sided hemiplegia, our duty of care is that we protect the left side … that's what we must do and provide all cares to make sure that there's no further damage occurs. But what we want to do for our residents is to make them feel good about the day by saying things like, 'Wow, isn't your right arm getting stronger now? Look, you're doing your exercises so well. Isn't it great the way you're standing on your leg? And look, you know, you're standing up straight. And oh, that's great and you're doing so well'. Because the thing that we can't take away from someone is hope and they must feel useful.

Families in denial

Because we've been in denial about ageing for so long, one of the spin-offs of that is that a lot … often the families are in denial about mum's dementia, the fact it's getting worse, the fact the person is approaching the end of their life and this is the end stage of a life span. Our society has been reluctant to hold open and frank discussions about this so often it's left up to the staff in the nursing home at the last minute to have the conversation with the families. And it can often be really distressing for the families because they have no experience about ageing and the last stages of life. And it's good to see that now there will be open discussions held about this is a normal part of … like birth and having children, going to school, they're all part of a life as is ageing and dying. We can't take one away from the other; it is part of a life process.

One of the things I often feel that the families would like me to be able to do and I say to them, 'I can do everything you want but I can't make your mum 20 years younger, I just can't do that. I know you would love to, I would love to but it just isn't anything that we can do'. And that's often a catalyst for them then to start to speak about, 'Well, what is going to happen now?' Because I think secretly somewhere they've been hoping that somebody could come up with this mystery wonderful answer that mum would be, or dad or husband or wife, would be fine if we just did this, if we just had a special diet or if we just had a special pill, if we just did something different that somehow or other we could reverse the ageing process. And I think sometimes that when you say the words that it can't be done, then that reality, you know, hits them and they then say, 'Well, where to from here?' So it's a great way to open it … I believe to start that conversation is, you know, 20 years younger but we can't do it. Yeah, so that's … it's really heartfelt to do that but, you know, sometimes it's the kind of way to introduce that end-of-life conversation.

Grief and loss

That's almost inherent in what we do now. We talk about it on admission, we have … I run grief and loss sessions, two probably a year, certainly one before Christmas where we mustn't assume that Christmas is a happy time for everybody. It's often very sad for people in an aged care facility if their families are all away, if they're the last one left in the family. If their spouse has passed away during the year and it's their first Christmas without them. So we hold grief and loss seminars in December, obviously, for the purpose of providing support during what is quite a traumatic time while everybody else is sort of trying to be jolly and it's a real conflicting set of emotions that you feel. So we are very sensitive to that and we do find that the staff spend a lot of time at the end of life talking to relatives about what they'd like. So we've had situations where people have been taken out … right up until the very last day have been taken to sit outside in the sunlight or in the light in the garden because that's where they love being. So you know, we can facilitate all of those sorts of things to make this the best experience that it can be. And perhaps we start talking about it being a celebration of a life well lived rather than looking at it as an entirely negative experience.

Death by inches

The people with their loved ones with the dementia have probably lost a lot of the contact with the person over the years. So for them it's more or less death by inches and it's, you know, they're often traumatised way before they realise that they've lost someone. So it could be … the last two years could have been just going through the motions of coming to visit, sitting with someone who's not responsive. And we work very hard on trying to retain connections—some connection—be it through … we had a music therapist and to maintain connections with that person so that there can be some quality of time spent with families in those later stages but we're not always successful. And when the people go I think sometimes it's a relief because they've let go of the person that they've loved as an entity and now they're just left with a physical being that doesn't resemble the person that they knew.

We're not the judges

And during this time some family members find it difficult to visit at all and we must … we have to support that and I think that's absolutely fine. You know, we're not the judges, we have no right to do that. We're there to support everybody and sometimes people feel more at peace with themselves if they didn't see someone they loved in those last few months when really the quality of life is fairly poor. So we respect everybody's choices at those times.

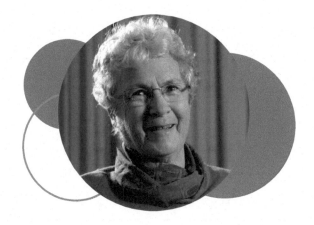

CHAPTER 10

Maureen's story

I'm Maureen Brady, and I'm now 74 years of age and I find as I get older, I reflect on my life and I think most people of my age do that.

I do find that some things I'm happy remembering, and some things are not so good, but the privilege of being older is that you can filter out what you don't want to remember.

Now, along the way I have married when I was 20. Had my family, four children.

When my family grew up, old enough for me to go back to work, I was involved with people who were ageing, people I had known in my home town. Then from there, my own mother started to age, and she was a very strong person, and I like to think that I have inherited her strengths. She was a wonderful woman, and her life hadn't been easy, but she was wonderful and positive always.

Changing my perspectives

Then the next part of my ageing experience was when my husband started to age. Then his health started to fail, and as that happened I had to readjust a lot of my thinking.

We moved for retirement, but from then on my husband's health was always an issue. So again, I was into changing my perspective, my needs, which as a mother, probably your needs back in those years went on hold, but then when it comes to your partner who you are expecting to support you when you get to that retirement time, when their health goes and you become once more the carer, I had already been the carer of my mother during her dying of cancer. So when I was caring for John at home, I enlisted the aid of first of all just housekeeping people. You have to let go of the fact that you are in charge, to a degree.

But along the way John's needs became greater, and he is now in care.

John moves into care

So again I had to adjust to this new lifestyle of having John in care and me visiting him.

Since John's been in care—he's been in care for 2½ years now—initially I wanted to be co-carer. I would be in here, I would be with him when the doctor came. I would be checking that he didn't have pain. Eventually after 2 years of doing that, we had a couple of crises, he nearly died just recently a second time, but my daughter came. I was not coping. Why? Because I was trying to continue to be carer, I was having difficulty letting go of that role. Now I visit him as his wife, not as his carer. I leave it to the staff of his caring facility to let me know when I am needed, why I'm needed, and I have a very good rapport with them. I've been able to let that co-carer—it hasn't been easy to do that, but I have managed. Now I come as his wife not as his carer.

Bloom where you are planted

We've been married 53 years. Now this is not at all what we expected our retirement to be like. We've retired in a lovely place, and there again, one of the sayings that I hang on to is, you bloom where you're planted. This is where I am, my family are an hour away, some of them are 3 hours away, but you connect with other people, and when you do that, it also shares—a trouble shared—but you do have to pick the people you do that with.

The other thing that I found is when speaking to people about my husband being in a nursing home, I hear lots of stories about my mother, when my mother was in a nursing home, when my father was in a nursing home, not too many stories about now my husband is in a nursing home. So that sort of does isolate you somewhat. Getting involved, I've got involved with a craft in his care community. The other people here, I've got involved in their stories, I've befriended some of them. Now it's lovely, it's a lovely feeling. So in my ageing I feel that I've been very blessed.

And I think positive thinking—you don't come by positive thinking easily though. You have to work at it, it's something you always have to work at. If you set yourself a goal, don't make it too difficult, make it just little things, even if it's to get the washing-up done today, and the bed made, that's big some days.

We need that contact

I always have a glass of red wine beside when my husband rings me at 6 o'clock every night on my mobile, because we need that contact. We need to have that goodnight. We've had it for all these years and we still do it. No matter where I am, I have my mobile on, and 6 o'clock, even the family, if we're sitting around together the family will say, 'It's 6 o'clock. That's Dad'.

Now John's in care … I had people say to me when John first came into care, directly from hospital, he never came home from that hospitalisation. They used to say, thank goodness you've done that, now you can get on with the rest of your life. Well, no; you can't. They are still here, and they still need your love and support, even though they don't show it. And the way they show it is different. Like if he knew I was here this morning, in his facility in another room, I have had to come and not let him know I'm here, because it's where's mum? If he knows I'm on the premises, if I get up to leave the room, where are you going? So I'm back … it's the cycle of life. I'm back to being the parent in a lot of ways. But still it's important and it's lovely, but it does not … if I have the opportunity to go and stay with family for three or four days for whatever purpose, I go knowing that John is in good care here. I still get the 6 o'clock phone calls.

A balanced life

Because you don't—you are so—you are very much into what other people need, and you have to have a balanced life. You've got to stick with the things that are important to you.

Well about my identity here, the staff if they want to address me, if I'm in one of the hallways, they'll call out 'John's wife'. My identity? What do you mean? So I'm identified as John's wife, and that's fine. Because I'm here every day I'm part of the furniture, but yeah, that's how they say, you know, they'll call me John's wife. Oh, that's John's wife over there, that's John's wife. John's wife's taught us to do that. <laugh> So that was funny.

In seeing your paperwork, something comes through the mail that used to come in John's name, now it comes in my name. And I'm thinking, oh … these are the moments when you get that insight into the fact that, yes, you are going to be on your own sooner or later. Well, that's not my decision, but the law of averages that's how it will happen. I try not to dwell on that.

Keeping him in the loop

So a part of keeping him in the circle, the phone, he can push a button and get either one of the children. The bottom one on the bottom row is my mobile, and he can ring me at 11 o'clock in the morning, just to say 'What are you doing?' So it's just keeping the lines of communication open, to whatever degree. He doesn't bother with the children so much now, because if you give him too much information too quickly, it confuses him.

So that continuity, he likes to hear funny little stories. They'll ring me and tell me, 'oh you can tell dad such and such'. So keep him in the loop, so to speak, to whatever degree. But the family are very aware of 'how are you doing, Mum', They're Very Good At That.

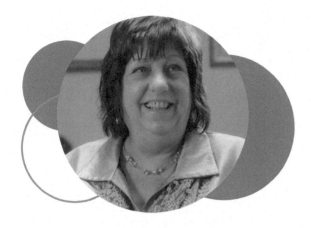

CHAPTER 10

Shirley's story

I've been a director of nursing in aged care since 1996. I've worked for for-profits, not-for-profits and government aged care facilities.

I can't change who they are

So I employ people based on the … who they are and do they fit the core values of the facility. So our core values are based on compassion, caring, honesty, integrity, respect for yourself, respect for others. Being, you know, kind, being fun, being, you know, so all the sorts of things we like in people who are going to have a positive impact when we meet them every day. Because I can educate a person and I can train them but I can't change their core values and I can't change who they are.

Power in relationships

The other thing about the residents is the way we speak to them. So if I'm coming in to shower someone, I would say to them, 'Can I help you with your shower now?' which, it doesn't sound a lot different from, 'I'm here to shower you now' but it has a huge impact on the power and the relationship. So when I say, 'Can I help you?' I'm allowing the resident to have the power to say, 'Look, I'm not ready yet' or 'I don't feel like it today' or 'I'd like to wear my pink dress' to have some interaction around it. When I make a statement like, 'I'm coming to shower you now', that's more or less a closed thing and the resident really doesn't have any power in that relationship. So all of this is how we train our carers and our staff to look at the way we provide care to our residents so that we're part of the team that, day-to-day, gets the best outcome every single day that that resident can expect, taking into account their physical and mental limitations.

Resident is the centre of care

The other thing that we're introducing, we're just working on now, is using the assessment to deliver care over a 24-hour continuum, not based around the tasks and the time that we do that group of tasks. So what we're doing now is like care mapping, so we take the assessments and we look at the time that the person may like to have a cup of tea at 3 o'clock in the morning. So rather than waiting for them to buzz, at 5 to 3 we make the cup of tea and we take it to them.

So what we're hoping to be able to do with all of these changes is to develop a care model where the resident is the centre of the care based on their assessed care needs about which we have a lot of information that we probably don't put to the very best use that we could. And having staff who respect the resident and work as part of the team of support workers around that resident for them to get the best they can out of their day, out of their quality of life. We have exercise classes every day and the numbers for that are just amazing. We're looking at putting in a gymnasium. We've got 106 volunteers here so we're very lucky with that. And they're all part of … we're really just a family or a community where we provide care around the residents. And they see a vibrant, active community all around them. And it makes them feel positive about every day they wake up, I hope. And that it's better than it could have been if had we continued in the old ways we used to do things.

Normalisation

We also are doing in our secure unit … we're looking at normalisation. So it's just something we're sort of looking at, at the moment is that we have a bus that goes out in the mornings and in the evenings and takes the residents for a short run, not very long, just … because when I asked them how old they were, they were somewhere between 20 and 50. And then we look at the behaviours and in the morning they're pacing and in the evening they're pacing even more. And when you think about what we're doing—what you were doing when you're between 20 and 50—you were going to work, going to school, going shopping and then you were coming back from school, coming back from shopping and coming back from work. So having and trying to replicate … trying to live in their reality, trying to replicate that lifestyle, for them to get in the bus and go to wherever it is they think their destination is and it doesn't really matter. And for them to be taken somewhere again in the afternoon, then this creates what they would consider to be their normal day, a normal pattern of a normal day for someone in that age group.

It's had a profound effect on negating a lot of the behaviours we were seeing in our residents. So they're more rested, they're more relaxed, they're not as anxious, they're not looking for, you know, 'where are the children?' and the things we do hear them say. So that's been absolutely wonderful because we can say—and they do remember because it happens five days a week—that yes, they've been out on the bus. And whatever the purpose of that journey was for them, then that's their reality.

I think that our customer base and their expectations will change dramatically over the next 5 to 10 years and beyond that as baby boomers come into the age care sector. They will expect that all of this will be in place, they will expect that their rights to make choices will be respected. They will expect that they will have access to the community, that they're not going to be isolated in the nursing home or the old people's home or that they won't see it like that.

Shared experiences

Look, they are so excited and once we start running with an idea I find they get super excited and then they … so some of them come on the bus trips every morning. So I've got one lady who comes in and goes on the bus twice a day with her sister because she likes to get out too. So there's just so much of that now that it's not … it becomes a shared experience for people. And that's just been wonderful because instead of it being us in control, the nursing staff in control of what happens to the residents' day, it's now a really shared experience getting the people in the bus out. They're seen by the community demystifies aged care. You know, we don't want to be placed, you know, up there on the hill where, you know, 'Oh, no, we don't go there'. So we want to remove all the stigmas and all the connotations because really ageing is just a part of life. It's a perfectly normal part of the process of a life span. So it's not to be denigrated, it's not to be feared, it's not to be, you know, if I stick my head in the sand, it won't catch up with me. So that by doing all of these things I believe that we'll take away the stigma and the mystery and the 'Oh, you know' about aged care and we'll be able to really share all our experiences with the community and then they'll come and share their experiences with us.